*Practice*
# Dentistry
# Pain-Free

## Evidence-Based Strategies
## to Prevent Pain and
## Extend Your Career

Bethany Valachi, PT, MS

Posturedontics Press
Portland, OR

Practice Dentistry Pain-Free: Evidence-Based Strategies to Prevent Pain and Extend Your Career

© 2008 Bethany Valachi

*Published by:*
Posturedontics Press
PO Box 25552
Portland, OR 97298
*www.posturedontics.com*

This book and related dental ergonomic products are available at: *www.posturedontics.com* or by calling 503-291-5121.

Editing by Matt Schlossberg
Cover design and interior by TLC Graphics, *www.TLCGraphics.com*
Illustrations by Janis Emerson
Graphics by TNT Graphics

ISBN: 978-0-9800778-0-3

1. Dental—Ergonomics—United States. 2. Dentistry—

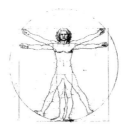

*My deepest thanks go to my husband, Keith, for his countless hours spent clinically testing various ergonomic interventions, dental ergonomic products and exercises.*
*His feedback, editorial suggestions and insights from a clinician's perspective have been an invaluable contribution to this book.*
*Keith's passion and dedication to this ergonomic education have helped make this book possible.*

———

Perhaps the most valuable result of all education is the

ability to make yourself do the thing you have to do,

when it ought to be done, whether you like it or not;

it is the first lesson that ought to be learned;

and however early a man's training begins,

it is probably the last lesson that he learns thoroughly.

THOMAS HENRY HUXLEY

———

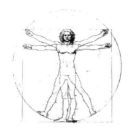

# Table of Contents

# Chapter 6: Dental Ergonomic Equipment . . . . . . . . .91

# Chapter 7: Operatory Layout and Systems . . . . . . .115

# Acknowledgements

The feedback and input from dozens of dental professionals, friends, and colleagues have contributed to the evolution of this book to its current state. I am deeply grateful:

To Keith and his dental team, who have tested various dental ergonomic equipment and graciously given up many a lunch hour for photo shoots: Kelly Mitts, Juli Muir, Tamra Dowdy, Marie Waite, Laura Cooper, Lori Spillman and Connie Paulson.

To my parents, for their love, encouragement and support of all my educational endeavors.

To my dear circle of girlfriends and my immediate family—the 'stabilizers' in my life that keep my priorities straight and keep me from taking myself, and life, too seriously.

To Linda Miles, my mentor, who has provided invaluable guidance in the development of an educational resource for dental professionals.

To my dental colleagues, Maxine Kane, Steve White, Steve Knight and Martha MacDonald, who have provided me with valuable education in each of their respective fields.

To Dr. Wayde Elliott, for his innovative titling of this book.

To Orlando Gomez, for his creative exercise photography and editing.

To my friends, colleagues and other professionals who have contributed their modeling talents for this book: Debbie Thorsness, Dawn Langnes, Orlando Gomez, Gayla Goodwin, Lacey Speed, Stephanie Keeler, Jennifer Craig, Dr. Manami Yamaguchi, Melissa McCoy, Raelene Wohlsen, Sandra Morris, Sandi Owen, Sherri Thompson, Cindy Kondrasky, Leslie Duclo, Ann Edlund, Kim Barbeau and Melissa Holm.

To the dental assistant instructors at OHSU School of Dentistry: Tammy Stange, Debra Hagg, Debra Sanchez and Kimberley Cummins.

To Lisa Rowley and Pacific University's School of Dental Hygiene for the use of their beautiful new facility.

To the following companies who have provided products that were used in photography: Orascoptic, Brewer, Scandex, Hager Worldwide, Perioptix, Smart Practice, Hu-Friedy, Crown Seating, Scrub Med and Pelton & Crane.

# Peer Reviewers

A special thank you to the following peer reviewers of this book for lending their time and expertise:

*Eric Shamus, PhD, MS, PT,* (co-author of Chapter 9), noted author and associate professor, College of Osteopathic Medicine, Nova Southeastern University, Fort Lauderdale, Florida

*David Ahearn, DDS,* president of Design Ergonomics Inc.

*Lance Rucker, DDS,* director of clinical simulation, University of British Columbia

*Dan O'Brien,* equipment specialist, Burkhart Dental, Portland, Oreg.

*Rene Cailliet, MD,* noted physiatrist and author of the "Pain Series"

*William B. Ericson, Jr., MD, FACS, FAAOS,* hand surgeon, Ericson Hand and Nerve Center, Seattle, Wash.

*Stacy Matsuda, RDH, BS,* Director of the Pacific NW Institute of periodontal therapy, Hillsboro, Oreg.

*John B. Nase, BS, DDS, FAGD, FICD,* author/lecturer, Harleysville, Penn.

*Maria Perno Goldie, RDH, MS,* editor-in-chief, *Modern Hygienist* journal

*Stuart McGill, PhD,* noted author and professor of spine mechanics at University of Waterloo, Canada

*Michael Fetzer,* president, Dental Systems Integrators Inc.

*Darlene Hertling, RPT, BS,* noted author and lecturer, Dept. of Rehabilitation Medicine, University of Washington School of Medicine, Seattle

*Timothy Welch, MS, DDS,* oral surgeon, Eugene, Oreg.

*Linda Thornton, DDS, MS,* associate professor, Temple University, Penn.

*John Ames, DDS,* oral surgeon, Spokane, Wash.

*Allan Jones, DDS,* general dentist and lecturer, Torrance, Calif.

*Kim Lierman, PT, ATC/R,* athletic trainer, Portland, Oreg.

# Disclaimer

This book is designed to provide information on injury prevention and is not intended to be a substitute for diagnosis or treatment of specific medical problems. The advice regarding preventive treatment, interventions and exercise is not suitable for everyone. Do not attempt self-diagnosis, and do not embark upon self-treatment of any kind without qualified medical supervision.

It is not the intention of this book to provide all information necessary in the prevention of pain and injuries in the dental profession, but rather to complement existing resources. The reader is urged to utilize the book's information and the Resources section at the end of this book, in conjunction with a healthcare professional, to develop an appropriate intervention program.

Every attempt has been made to provide the latest and most accurate information, studies and references. However, there may be errors or omissions; therefore, this text should be used only as a general guide.

Nothing in this book should be construed as a promise of benefits or of results to be achieved, or a guarantee by the author or publisher of the safety or efficacy of its contents. The author, Posturedontics LLC, and the publisher shall have neither liability nor responsibility to any person or entity with respect to any loss, injury or damage caused, or alleged to have been caused directly or indirectly by the information contained in this book.

If you do not wish to be bound by the above disclaimer, please return your copy of the book to the publisher for a full refund.

# Preface–Note to Reader

Occupational pain in dentistry is a chronic problem that can adversely affect your career, leisure activities, personal lifestyle and income. As a physical therapist married to a dentist, I had a personal as well as a financial interest in shedding light on this problem. It is my sincere hope that this book will help you and countless others enjoy a comfortable and long career in the profession for which you have so diligently trained.

This book is intended for both dentists and hygienists, with special chapters devoted to assistants and front office. It is organized so that you can easily turn to a desired chapter, such as Chapter 4 on neck pain. (*It is recommended that you read Chapters 1 and 2 before proceeding to any of the other chapters.*) Keep in mind, when reading the chapters that target specific body areas, the interconnectedness of the human body. For instance, certain strategies in the low-back section may also benefit the neck. Not all areas of the body are included, due to constraint of book size. Therefore, this additional education will be available via electronic newsletters and special articles at *www.posturedontics.com*.

This volume is meant not only for individuals experiencing chronic pain, but just as important, for dental professionals and new graduates who are purchasing ergonomic equipment, interested in preventing pain and ensuring an optimal quality of life.

While ergonomic advice is abundant in various dental educational formats, I have observed a general lack of understanding and education as to *how* dental ergonomic equipment, adjustment, operatory layouts, delivery systems, postures and positioning impact the dental professional's musculoskeletal health.

There seems to be a gap of knowledge between the science of dental ergonomics and the associated work-related pain. It's time to bridge that gap.

*Bethany Valachi*
Portland, Oregon

# CHAPTER ONE

---

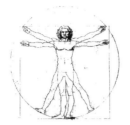

# The Journey Begins

An ounce of prevention is worth a pound of cure.

BEN FRANKLIN

"Geez, Beth, my back is killing me!" My husband, Keith, had returned from work at his dental practice. Not exactly the lyrical "Honey, I'm home" I had anticipated.

"I'm ready to sell that practice," he said. "I can't go on working in pain like this—it feels like a knife in the middle of my back.

"Can you work on my back again tonight?" he asked. "Maybe another massage or mobilization would help."

So began another evening of what was becoming the norm for our relationship.

Does this sound familiar to you? Not only are dental professionals affected by work-related pain, but frequently there is a negative impact on their families and social lives.

One would think that marriage to a physical therapist would be a godsend. This illusion was short-lived. Keith soon came to realize that during his massage euphoria I was devising a prevention plan that would enable him to self-treat and prevent his own pain. I went to his office and analyzed his posture and body mechanics in the operatory; this is where the intervention really needed to start. Using this information, I developed a prevention plan that included new postural, positioning and exercise techniques. Keith's pain began to resolve.

Eight years later, he still practices dentistry full time. Although he continues to face intermittent musculoskeletal challenges that are a reality for nearly all dental professionals, his chronic low-back pain is gone. The nightly massages stopped years ago.

Helping Keith learn to manage his chronic low-back pain raised my interest in the problem and prompted me to research the topic. What I learned is startling. The prevalence of musculoskeletal pain, disorders and disability is alarmingly high in the dental profession. An average of two out of three dental care workers experience pain.[1-18]

I also discovered a gap of knowledge in the literature. On the one hand, there were dental ergonomic experts who advised on the selection, adjustment and use of equipment and operatory layouts. On the other hand, there were healthcare professionals who explored symptoms of musculoskeletal disorders among dental professionals. What was missing was a link between the two. How do certain chair adjustments promote specific pain syndromes? How do different operatory layouts cause movement patterns that lead to other pain syndromes? What chairside working positions cause the muscle imbalances typically seen among dental professionals?

These, and many other questions, changed the direction of my career—from clinical physical therapist to dental ergonomist. I spent years researching the topic, became a certified ergonomic assessment specialist, then began providing dental ergonomic consultations and seminars. What I discovered is that this missing information is actually what many team members were looking for. I soon realized that my background, combined with Keith's clinical experience and his staff's willingness to participate in evaluating equipment and implementing research-based preventive strategies, was a winning combination for raising this education to a new level.

Today, I am still fascinated with the unique challenges the dental team faces and humbled by the vast expanse of knowledge in biomechanics, kinesiology, physiology, dental ergonomics and equipment technologies required to effectively address the problem of occupational pain and disability among dental professionals.

However, my research and clinical experiences have convinced me that there is hope and promise that the profession can effectively decrease the high incidence of pain among dental operators. I believe that accurate education, combined with implementation of appropriate strategies and proper equipment selection and modification can significantly reduce and prevent work-related pain. It also can help *you* identify and treat your own pain and discomfort *before* it becomes severe enough to require medical attention.

Even those who continue to practice in pain after receiving medical treatment may benefit from understanding what the preponderance of research has revealed and how it can be applied in clinical dentistry. Unfortunately, recent dental-school graduates, many of whom have yet to experience work-related pain, embrace the "it could never happen to me" mindset—they take few ergonomic precautions until

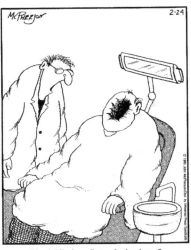

"You let that cavity go far too long."

CLOSE TO HOME © 1995 John McPherson. Reprinted with permission of UNIVERSAL PRESS SYNDICATE. All rights reserved.

the painful episode occurs. Years later, I often hear these same individuals say, "I wish I had paid more attention earlier in my career," or "In dental school I thought I was invincible. I didn't realize the magnitude of this problem in our profession."

So, if you are a dentist, hygienist or student who is interested in optimizing your musculoskeletal health, becoming savvy with equipment selection, operating more comfortably or extending your career, this book is for you.

Numerous studies have been conducted on the prevalence of work-related pain in dentistry.[1-19] The results indicate that more than half of all practicing dental professionals experience work-related pain. This pain often begins in dental[20] or hygiene school.[21] More than 70 percent of dental students complain of musculoskeletal pain by their third year.[20] Among hygiene students, nearly 37 percent report neck pain; however, the prevalence is higher among hygienists who have previously worked as assistants.[21] Keith was one of the unfortunate individuals whose musculoskeletal pain began at this early stage of his career.

It is clear from the research that the delivery of dental care poses potentially significant risks of injury to practitioners. Now that the problem has been established, the crucial next step is ascertaining exact causes, then researching and developing effective prevention strategies.

From a compilation of numerous studies on pain, we can see that each dental team member is predisposed to pain or injury in slightly different areas of the body, depending on his or her tasks and positioning relative to the patient.

For example, hygienists are predisposed to a higher incidence of neck, shoulder and hand/wrist pain[2] largely due to static postures combined with forceful, repetitive movements inherent to the job. Oral surgeons are more prone to leg pain, probably due to standing work postures, while endodontists complain more of arm and shoulder pain likely due to forceful arm movements.[8] General dentists, on the other hand, tend to be more susceptible to lower back injuries, largely due to prolonged static postures (PSPs).[22]

Unlike most manufactured products, you didn't arrive in this world with a bag of spare parts. You have what you have, and you must take care of it. While the occasional mild back or neck ache is not cause for alarm, if regularly occurring pain or discomfort is ignored, the cumulative physiological damage can lead to a career-ending injury or cumulative trauma disorder (CTD). Unfortunately, occupational pain comes with not only a physical cost, but a significant financial burden as well.

# Impact on Productivity and Profitability

In 1987, the estimated loss in income due to musculoskeletal pain in dentistry was $41 million.[18] In 2004, the average general dentist worked about 200 days, netting $930 per day.[23] If dentists lost only one day per year due to musculoskeletal pain, as in Shugars' 1987 study, the annual income lost in general dentistry due to musculoskeletal pain in 2004 was approximately $131 million.

Nearly 30 percent of all dentists who retire early are forced to do so due to a musculoskeletal disorder.[24] In 2004, one insurance company paid more than $24.6 million in cash benefits to American Dental Association (ADA) members who became disabled after November 1, 1992.[25] Of those dentists on claim in 2004, 14 percent were dentists disabled on or before age 45.[25] To get an idea of the direct impact of CTDs, imagine if a dentist is forced to retire only five years early; the lost wages could easily be more than $1 million. Additionally, employers' worker's compensation premiums may increase as a result of employees' claims.

Financial losses can also be significant for dental hygienists whose wages range from $25 to $50 per hour, with the average being $32.50 per hour.[26] Although losing a single day of work costs hygienists one day's wages, few hygienists who sustain a CTD lose only one workday. Many miss weeks or months, or they retire early.[27] Numerous dental hygienists reduce the number of days they work due to work-related pain. One in five hygienists who permanently leave the profession is affected by a disability.[28] Due to the physically demanding nature of practicing as a clinical dental hygienist, short and long term disabilities are common, thus, few disability insurance companies are willing to take the risk of protecting the income for those in the dental hygiene profession.[27]

Consider how a dental hygienist with poor musculoskeletal health also can adversely impact a practice's bottom line:

- *Loss of productivity* – Between $800 and $1,400 per day of practice income can be lost.

- *Restorative treatment* – Consider that a majority of the practice's restorative treatment scheduling comes out of the hygiene department.

- *Goodwill* – While some practices may view staff as expendable, patients do not like to see turnover. Goodwill may be affected if you must continually cancel appointments due to a hygienist's ill-health.

- *Temporary* – Utilizing a temporary hygienist may result in altered quality of care since the hygienist is not familiar with the patient, and temporaries may be less inclined to recommend treatment to patients.

# Cumulative Trauma Disorders

Perhaps nowhere is the literature more confusing than when it comes to defining dysfunction of the musculoskeletal system. The alphabet soup of acronyms describes virtually the same thing: musculoskeletal disorder (MSD), repetitive strain injury (RSI), repetitive motion injury (RMI), repetitive trauma injury (RTI), cumulative trauma disorder (CTD) or overuse syndrome (OUS).

In dentistry, such disorders usually begin as microtrauma: microscopic damage that occurs to certain parts of your musculoskeletal system on a daily basis.[22] Your body is well equipped to deal with this damage and is constantly repairing this microtrauma when your body is at rest. In dentistry, however, rest breaks are often insufficient. The rate of damage to your body accumulates faster than the body can repair it. Microtrauma occurs on a cellular level, and the damage is cumulative. You often don't feel any discomfort until enough tissue damage accumulates that pain and muscle dysfunction occur; a pain syndrome is born. Since this accumulation mechanism best describes how injuries develop in dentistry, the term cumulative trauma disorder (CTD) will be used throughout this book. CTDs are theorized to be the primary cause of disability among dentists, hygienists and assistants. If not attended to early, CTDs may lead to acute injury, chronic pain syndromes or permanent disability. The damaged tissue eventually becomes painful and inflamed, resulting in loss of function.

Warning signs and symptoms of a CTD include: decreased strength, such as gripping strength on a dental instrument; decreased range of motion, such as turning your head to look over your shoulder while driving home; pain or burning; numbness or tingling sensations; shooting or stabbing pain, usually into an arm or leg; and swelling or inflammation.

The most common CTDs in dentistry are:

- *Chronic low-back pain.* Pain in the low back or shooting pain/numbness into the hip, buttock or one leg. This may be due to muscle spasm, trigger points, spinal disc degeneration or herniation, facet joint inflammation or numerous other etiologies. In dentistry, low-back pain is often caused by poor seated posture and weak stabilizing trunk muscles.

- *Tension neck syndrome.* Pain, stiffness, muscle hardening, trigger points and tenderness in the neck musculature, occiput, between the shoulder blades, and sometimes numbness or tingling in one arm or hand. In dentistry, a common cause is forward head posture.

- *Trapezius myalgia.* Pain, tenderness, trigger points and muscle hardening in the upper trapezius muscle due to sustained contraction of the muscle. Risk factors in dentistry include chronic elevation of the shoulders and emotional tension.

- *Rotator cuff impingement.* Pain in the shoulder upon overhead reaching, sustained arm elevation or sleeping on the affected arm. Operating with abducted arm posture is a major risk factor.

- *Carpal tunnel syndrome.* Pain, numbness or tingling into the hand and fingers usually due to compression of the median nerve in the carpal tunnel of the wrist. Numerous risk factors are involved, including flexed wrist posture, instruments with small diameters, gender and forceful grip.

To prevent CTDs and maintain optimal musculoskeletal health, the cause of your work-related pain must be understood. You should learn the unique muscle imbalances to which you are prone and how various work postures, positions, adjustment of ergonomic equipment and exercise can positively or negatively affect your personal musculoskeletal health.

# What's Causing Your Pain?

Musculoskeletal pain stems from numerous sources, including genetic predisposition, environment, previous injuries and age. While you have little control over these factors, you do have control over other work-related causes of MSDs, including prolonged static postures, repetitive movements, suboptimal lighting, patient/operator positioning, mental stress, physical conditioning and poor or improperly adjusted ergonomic equipment. (Fig. 1)

## Fig. 1: Risk factors leading to CTDs in dentistry

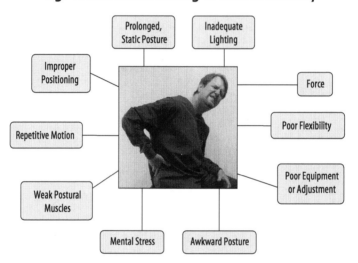

If ignored, these risk factors can promote structural damage in the body. This damage begins as microtrauma, or cellular-level damage that occurs on a daily basis. It may continue unnoticed for months or even years before enough microtrauma builds up to elicit pain.

It would be easy to just tell you how to sit, position yourself, which equipment to buy and which exercises to perform. However, to obtain lasting and profound changes in your health, you need to understand *why* you're making these changes.

Once we lay this foundation of understanding, you will not only understand the reasoning behind the recommendations in this book, you also will be able to make informed decisions regarding equipment selection, therapies, nutrition, sports and other daily activities.

One risk factor in particular that leads to significant physiological damage in dentistry is prolonged static postures (PSPs).[22] This microtrauma develops through a series of events. (Fig. 2)

# Microtrauma from Prolonged Static Postures

The human body was designed for movement. Over tens of thousands of years, the human body has depended on movement for its survival. But industrial and technological advances have done much to impede Mother Nature. With the onset of the Industrial Revolution, increasing numbers of workers perform relatively stationary tasks. With the advent of computers the number of sedentary jobs has increased. So too have the number of CTDs, resulting in the formation of organizations such as the Occupational Safety and Health Administration (OSHA) and the National Institute for Occupational Safety and Health (NIOSH) in 1970.

One study showed the prevalence of low-back pain has increased by 2,700 percent from 1980 to 1993.[29] It is reasonable to infer that changes in the way we use our bodies has contributed to this dramatic increase in work-related pain. In short, the body must move—and move properly—to stay healthy.

**Fig. 2: Flowchart showing how prolonged static postures can progress to pain or a CTD**

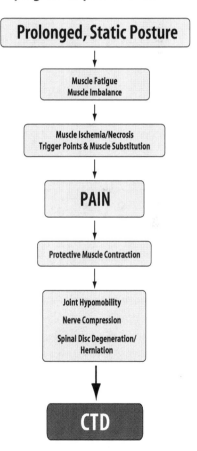

9

A similar change has occurred since the introduction of four-handed dentistry—dentists tend to work for longer periods of time without taking a break, and they perform longer procedures.[11] Consider that when you sit in a static operating posture without leaning on your chair's backrest, more than 50 percent of your body's muscles must contract to hold the body motionless while resisting gravity. The static forces resulting from these PSPs are much more taxing on the body than dynamic (moving) forces.[13] It isn't just prolonged sitting that causes such problems. Assuming any posture for prolonged periods of time can overwork soft tissues and promote pain syndromes.[30] The resultant microtrauma from these PSPs include muscle imbalances, muscle ischemia, trigger points and spinal disc degeneration.

## *Muscle imbalances*

Dentists, hygienists and assistants should ideally strive to maintain a neutral, balanced posture. However, even with the best ergonomic equipment, dental operators frequently find themselves leaning or twisting, usually more in one direction than the other. For example, most right-handed dentists tend to lean forward and to the *right* when they leave their neutral operating posture.[31] Over time, the muscles can adaptively shorten on one side of the body, spine or joint.[32] (Fig. 3) This imbalance can exert asymmetrical forces, causing misalignment of the spinal column or joints, with loss of range of motion in one direction over the other.

**Fig 3: Adaptive muscle shortening can lead to a plethora of pain syndromes**

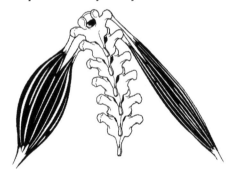

You can test for this imbalance yourself: If you are a right-handed operator, side-bend your neck to the left and rotate your head to the right. Now perform this on the opposite side. Does one side feel tighter than the other? Most right-handed dentists repeatedly side-bend the neck to the right and rotate the neck to the left to gain better visibility, which results in more flexibility in this direction, but increased stiffness in the opposite direction.[16] I have observed that by only their sixth month of dental or hygiene school, muscle imbalances are present in most students. In Chapters 3 and 4, we will explore specific muscle imbalances in greater depth.

Perhaps even more common among dental professionals are postural muscle imbalances that develop between the stabilizer muscles and the mover muscles of the body. A common pattern involves shortening and tightening of certain mover muscles and weakening of stabilizer muscles.[33] (Chapter 4) Over time, the body's musculature can adapt to the abnormal posture caused by these muscle imbalances and tend to maintain this unbalanced posture not only at work, but in leisure activities as well.[32]

## Muscle ischemia

Maintaining static postures in dentistry requires sustained muscle contraction. When a muscle is contracted for a prolonged period of time, intramuscular pressure rises. This pressure compresses the blood vessels within the muscle, and during strong static contractions, can almost completely obstruct blood flow through the muscle.[34] As lactic acid accumulates, muscular pain and fatigue result.[34,35,36] Dentists and hygienists perform *static muscle work* frequently, for example, when holding an instrument. *Dynamic muscle work*, on the other hand, creates a healthier environment for bodily repair. (Fig. 4) The rhythmic, pump-like contraction and relaxation of the muscles ensures adequate blood flow and oxygen to the muscles, as well as lactic acid removal. Roving assistants perform dynamic muscle work, such as walking, cleaning treatment rooms and preparing instrument trays, throughout their day. Their pain frequency is typically below that of the rest of the team.

Even in the most neutral working postures, your body must still maintain static muscle contractions. And when your posture deviates from neutral, the muscles must contract even harder to maintain upright working posture. As muscles fatigue, this prolonged contraction can cause muscle ischemia.[36]

**Fig. 4: Dynamic muscle work delivers more blood to muscles than static work**

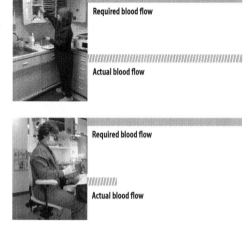

Recovery time is relatively rapid after brief periods of high-level-intensity muscle work, such as 20 minutes of uphill bicycling. However, recovery time from low-level muscle fatigue after working a seven- to eight-hour day (as in dentistry) is much longer. There is a risk that muscles may not even recover by the following workday. Human muscles are not designed for continuous, long-lasting contractions. They require rest periods to recover from even low-level exertion.[37]

It is a physiologic certainty that if the rate of tissue damage exceeds the rate of repair due to insufficient rest periods, muscle necrosis can result. As more tissue within a certain muscle becomes damaged, the body may call upon another muscle entirely to perform a job for which it was not designed, a concept known as muscle substitution. An abnormal, "compensatory" motion may then develop and predispose the person to a myriad of musculoskeletal dysfunctions.

## *Trigger points*

If you are a dentist or hygienist, you are probably already painfully aware of trigger points. A trigger point is a group of muscle fibers that is in a constant state of contraction. (Fig. 5) It feels like a hard knot, nodule or small pea. When pressed upon, it may be painful locally or refer pain to a distant part of the body. It neither allows the muscle to contract, nor relax, thereby effectively decreasing flexibility and range of motion. A trigger point may be active (painful) or latent (causing stiffness and restricting range of motion). Because they are caused by prolonged muscle contraction, postural asymmetry and mental stress, it is easy to see why trigger points are so common among dental professionals. Ischemic muscles are especially susceptible to the development of trigger points.[38]

If allowed to persist untreated, some trigger points can cause compression on nerves and contribute to syndromes such as thoracic outlet syndrome or pronator teres syndrome (a carpal tunnel-type pain). Since many trigger points are caused by postural asymmetry, specific operatory modifications are frequently necessary to prevent their recurrence.

**Fig. 5: A trigger point is actually comprised of many smaller muscle fiber contractions**

(Travell, Simons, *Myofascial Pain and Dysfunction: The trigger point manual.* Edited, EP Johnson, Wilkins & Wilkins 1999. Reproduced with permission.)

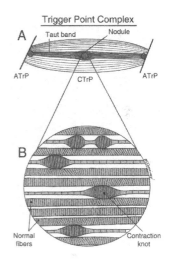

Painful trigger points are not only common among dental professionals; they also can afflict your patients. Trigger points in the masseter, temporalis or pterygoid muscles may cause a "muscular toothache," which may be misdiagnosed or referred to a specialist if the dentist is not knowledgeable of these referral patterns.[38] Self-treatment of trigger points will be discussed in Chapter 8.

## *Final progression to a CTD*

Once microtrauma causes pain, the body often initiates a protective muscle contraction, or spasm, to immobilize the area and prevent further injury. This is usually the symptom of an underlying problem, not the cause.[32] Unfortunately, this frequently leads to more problems such as compression on nerves, tendonitis, joint stiffness and spinal disc herniation. Once you develop a CTD, you are at a much higher risk for a recurrence of a similar musculoskeletal problem in the future. Therefore, the importance of prevention cannot be overstated. Without appropriate intervention, these physiological changes can, over time, lead to discomfort or pain—even the end of your career.

# Treat the Cause or Treat the Effect?

In a society that demands instant gratification, it is tempting to lean toward quick fixes such as pain medication or surgery. However, treatments that are oriented toward immediate relief are also often temporary. It's not that treatments aren't effective in the short term; it's that you are often returning to the habits and positions that caused the pain in the first place. Therefore, addressing work habits and environment are a good first step in effectively preventing and managing pain syndromes.

## *Ergonomics*

Put simply, ergonomics is the science of fitting jobs to the people who work them. The goal of an ergonomics program is to improve worker performance and reduce occupational pain and injuries by modifying work areas and equipment to reduce damaging postures, positions and body motions. As it applies to dentistry, ergonomics involves the design, adjustment and modification of operatory layouts, counters, delivery systems, stools, instruments and patient chairs to minimize excessive reaching, twisting, leaning, gripping and repetitive motions. In addition to workplace modification, dental operators should be educated on proper body mechanics and preventive exercise to safeguard against injuries.

Dental ergonomic solutions have historically been mostly equipment-based or protocol-based. Equipment-based solutions have the obvious problem of bias. It is sometimes difficult to get an unbiased or objective assessment of a product's effectiveness from a sales representative. Protocol-based education may be grounded in past institutional practices. For example, you may have been taught to operate in specific positions or to sit a certain "correct" way. Sometimes, however, there is little or no supportive research as to how these protocols and positions impact your musculoskeletal health or why following such advice would benefit you.

My thesis advisor in graduate school taught me a valuable lesson regarding interpreting information and scientific studies—he said, "Question everything." Sage advice, indeed. I feel it is imperative that dental professionals "separate the wheat from the chaff" by requesting supportive evidence for ergonomic claims or advice. You should be able to obtain answers to questions like, "How is this patient positioning affecting my shoulder joint?" or "How does this chair height affect my lumbar spine?"

The answers to these kinds of questions must be evidence-based and readily available to ensure that following such advice will actually benefit you.

## *Ergonomics education*

In light of the prevalence of pain among students and the high disability rate among practicing dentists and hygienists, it is imperative that ergonomics and musculoskeletal wellness education begin in school. Dr. Albert Guay of the American Dental Association (ADA) advises that ergonomic practices should be incorporated into initial training programs.[39] Studies in Europe make similar recommendations for ergonomic training based on the prevalence of pain among their dental student population. The results of an unpublished ADA survey found that 62 percent of private practice dentists felt they received inadequate training in ergonomics in dental school.[39] An assessment on ergonomic education in dental hygiene schools found that while a majority offered basic education in operator/patient positioning and instrumentation, additional education (body mechanics, preventive exercise) was unavailable.[42]

Due to dental care workers' predisposition to unique muscle imbalances, ischemia and trigger points, an effective dental ergonomics education program for both schools and practicing dental professionals should include specialized education in several areas:

- *Biomechanics.* The external forces acting upon the operator's body parts due to operatory layout, equipment and environment. A study on the need for dental ergonomics training in dental schools pointed specifically to hiring individuals who are trained in the application of biomechanics.[43]

- *Kinesiology.* This is how certain movements you make in the operatory impact specific joints and muscles. Without this knowledge, you are blindly adopting the shotgun approach to pain prevention and management. This is the "missing link" in much ergonomic education.

- *Anatomy/physiology.* You need to have a basic understanding of how your body functions to understand how movements, equipment features and adjustments impact your health. More attention needs to be given as to how gender differences impact dental professionals.

- *Dental equipment knowledge.* Today's market has a plethora of constantly evolving and changing dental ergonomic equipment. Keeping current on these developments requires significant time investment.

- *Dental equipment adjustment.* It is not enough to simply recommend dental ergonomic equipment such as dental magnification loupes. Specific guidelines for selection, adjustment and measurements are needed, in addition to *how* factors impact the operator's musculoskeletal health. For instance, improper measurement of the operator's working distance on a new pair of $1,200 loupes can actually worsen neck pain.

- *Dental equipment modification.* Wouldn't it be nice to know if there were modifications you could make to your existing $13,000 patient chair instead of buying a new one? Options should be provided for retrofitting existing equipment to make "ergonomizing" your operatory more economical.

- *Preventive exercise.* Unique muscle imbalances and strength requirements should be addressed with chairside stretching and specific exercises to develop balanced musculoskeletal health. Dentists and hygienists should also be educated on which exercises may cause worsening of their musculoskeletal health and pain syndromes.

## ERGONOMIC BENEFITS

The benefits of implementing ergonomic and injury prevention techniques into your daily routine can have a profound impact for dental professionals, including:

- Managed and reduced musculoskeletal pain
- Prevention of work-related injuries
- Increased energy levels and productivity
- Decreased job stress
- Improved employee morale and decreased employee turnover
- Decreased number of sick days and a safer workplace
- Improved quality of life and job satisfaction
- Increased career longevity

# Prevention: The Best Health Insurance

It seems to be human nature to address musculoskeletal issues only when they become acutely painful, with little attention to the source of the problem.

In the United States, less than 5 cents out of every healthcare dollar is spent on public-health research.[44] Fortunately, this trend is slowly reversing as more businesses and insurance companies recognize the physical and financial benefits of research that leads to effective prevention programs.

Customized, in-office ergonomic intervention programs are becoming more popular, as they have been shown to effectively

## Fig. 6: Dental Patients—Prevention or Pain?

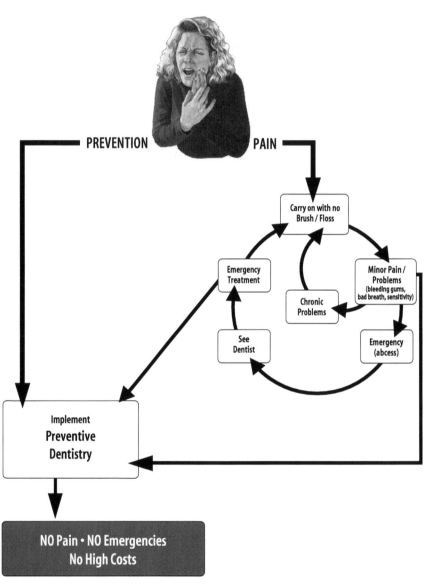

© 2000 Posturedontics

## Fig. 7: Dental Professionals—Prevention or Pain?

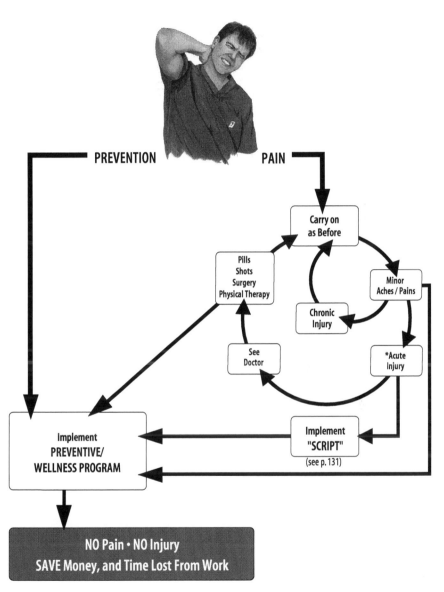

reduce workers' pain symptoms, increase productivity, decrease lost workdays and more. A personalized ergonomic intervention program, *combined with* ergonomic education, has been shown to be significantly more effective at reducing worker musculoskeletal symptoms when compared with ergonomic education alone.[45] After an ergonomic intervention in the Netherlands, 72 percent of dentists reported a reduction or resolution of their main physical complaint.[46] Implementation of an early intervention, work training and job re-design program at American Biltrite, Inc. resulted in a 90 percent reduction in back injury claims and a 50 percent reduction in lost workdays.[32] Other studies reveal reductions of up to 81 percent of physical problems through ergonomic intervention programs,[47] as well as fewer lost workdays and decreased worker's compensation expenses.[48-52] Among my dental ergonomic consulting clients, 77 percent of team members have reported decreased pain at three months post-consultation.

It behooves dentists and hygienists to seek coverage from disability and insurance companies that are proactive from a prevention standpoint and offer specific dental ergonomic education, rather than waiting for their insured to become injured before taking action.

You instruct your patients in preventive oral healthcare so they can enjoy good oral health for their lifetime. (Fig. 6) Shouldn't you also adopt the same philosophy for your own musculoskeletal health? (Fig. 7)

With this foundation of knowledge established, you will now have a better understanding of the reasoning behind the evidence-based strategies presented in this text. Let's now take the next step on your journey toward improved musculoskeletal health as we explore the *Three P's to Fitness* in the operatory.

# CHAPTER TWO

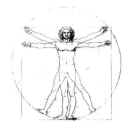

# The 3 P's to Fitness in the Operatory:
## Posture, Positioning and Periodic Stretching

---

Make it a point to do something every day
that you don't want to do. This is the golden rule
for acquiring the habit of doing your duty without pain.

---

MARK TWAIN

o maintain musculoskeletal wellness in dentistry, it is helpful to understand three basic concepts that impact every part of your body. First, every part of your body has a neutral posture. This is the position in which the least amount of stress is placed on the muscles, nerves, ligaments, tendons and joints. For example, neutral posture of the head is ear-over-shoulder when viewed from the side.

Second, you must understand the need for a variety of positioning strategies to attain neutral postures. A single strategy won't work because several factors are at play, including the size of your patients, their tolerance to supine positioning, operator size and patient chair design.

---

Third, you must understand how periodic stretching and movement can counter the microtrauma imposed upon your body from unavoidable daily prolonged static postures. (Chapter 1)

In the next three chapters I'll describe how each of these concepts applies to specific areas of your body. Here, I'll show you why these concepts matter.

# Postural Awareness

Posture is a product of numerous inputs throughout your life. Genetics, self-impression, attitude, conditioning and occupation all impact how you hold your body. If you were tall, had large breasts or a poor self-image when growing up, you may have developed a slumped posture that your body has perceived as "normal." If there was no discomfort, this posture may have been carried into adulthood. Likewise, in an occupation like dentistry, your head is usually in a slight degree of forward posture, even when wearing loupes. Over time, your suboccipital muscles may adaptively shorten to hold your head in this poor posture. This is an example of *muscle adaptation*.[1] Your brain may now perceive that 20 degrees of forward head posture is normal, or good head posture. This is known as altered *proprioception*.[2] You may not even realize the postural change, since there may be few warning signs until significant microtrauma is sustained. (Chapter 1)

Due to these postural events, discovering your own optimal posture through proprioception may not be effective for many practicing dental professionals and students. Poor working postures are readily observed among dental and hygiene students. By their third year in dental school more than half of these students experience neck pain,[3] which can cause poor neck proprioception.[4] This lack of proprioception also increases with *frequency* of neck pain.[5] The proprioceptive model may work well for entry-level dental students and for those practicing dental professionals who have not developed postural dysfunction and/or pain syndromes.

Poor posture accelerates wear and tear on your vertebrae, discs, muscles and ligaments and can lead to multiple pain syndromes.[2,6] It decreases your lung capacity and oxygen intake,[2] which is vital to your musculoskeletal health; causes muscle imbalances that can lead to CTDs like thoracic outlet syndrome;[7,8] and can impair sleep patterns. Consider that poor posture also can make you look older, shorter and heavier.

On the other hand, good postural habits can positively impact your health, recreational activities and career longevity. Due to the significant postural demands of dentistry, the importance of incorporating these concepts into your life are greatly magnified. A conscious effort must therefore be made by dental professionals to defray the damaging postural effects of their occupations. This must become a *lifestyle habit* that is carried outside the operatory, into the home, onto the golf course and into all your activities, including sleep.

A basic primer on anatomy and physiology will help you understand how damage occurs in various seated and standing operator postures and how different equipment affects musculoskeletal health. Let's start with the spine, which has four natural curves when viewed from the side: the cervical lordosis, thoracic kyphosis, lumbar lordosis and sacral kyphosis.[1] Since the sacral curve is comprised of five fused vertebrae, its movement is extremely limited. However, the remaining curves are more mobile and therefore influenced by their neighboring curves. (Fig. 1) The spinal curves are interdependent. Change in any one curve will result in a change in the curve above or below it.[9] As mentioned previously, the degree of these curves (your posture) is based on emotional, occupational and genetic factors.[6]

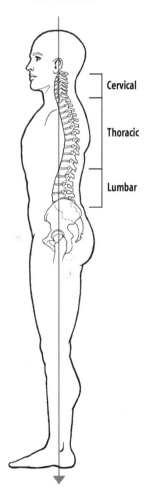

**Fig. 1: The three movable curves of the human spine: cervical, thoracic and lumbar**

Cervical

Thoracic

Lumbar

In neutral spinal posture, the curves of your spine are all present and balanced, and the spine is supported mostly by the bony structure of the vertebrae resting on top of one another, resulting in minimal strain on muscles and surrounding tissue. Occupational challenges may cause you to work in positions that flatten or exaggerate the spinal curves. This can distort your sense of neutral posture and result in muscle imbalances that cause the spine to depend increasingly on muscles, ligaments, and soft tissue to remain erect. These tissues gradually adapt to the postural deformity and begin to hold the body in improper alignment when working inside and outside the operatory. (Fig. 2)

### Fig. 2: Variations in spinal posture.
### Note how the low-back curve affects the other spinal curves

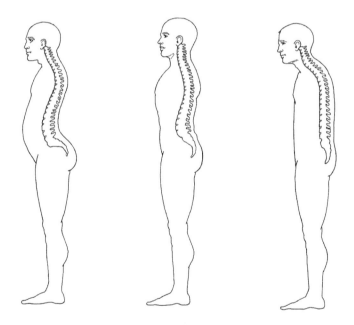

The spine serves multiple functions in your body. It houses and protects your spinal cord; provides a rigid structure to resist gravity, allowing an upright posture; and allows your body to move. This spinal flexibility is achieved through a series of alternating bony vertebrae and spinal discs. The bony vertebrae protect the spinal cord and nerves—the electrical powerhouse of the body. Between each vertebra is the spinal disc, which acts as a shock absorber and allows you to bend, twist and lean. Inside each disc is the gel-like nucleus. Surrounding the nucleus are diagonally oriented layers of tough fibrous collagen fibers, which hold the nucleus inside the disc. Each layer of diagonal fibers is opposite the underlying layer, similar to a wicker basket. Hence, they are well suited to resist a straight-down compressive force but are susceptible to damage by twisting forces.[10]

Neutral standing posture is ear, shoulder, hip and ankle in alignment when viewed from the side. (Fig. 1) In this standing posture, the pelvis is at an angle that optimally supports and balances the spine and minimizes muscular exertion. The spine is supported primarily by the bony vertebral structure and the posterior vertebral facets. In seated dentistry, however, your sitting posture tends to disengage the facets and transfer the load to the discs.[11] Therefore, seated dentistry may place the operator at a greater risk for disc damage than standing dentistry. (However, standing dentistry imposes other musculoskeletal strain.) The challenge of maintaining balanced spinal curves becomes greatly magnified in the seated position.

# Operator Posture

## *Position yourself first*

Due to anthropometric differences, ideal seated posture will vary slightly between dental operators; however, it is important to define an accurate ergonomic reference posture from which to start. To attain neutral seated posture, you should have a slight curve in the low back, shoulders over hips, elbows relaxed at the sides and forearms approximately parallel with the floor.[11,12] Neutral head posture is ears-over-shoulder when viewed from the side; however, this ideal posture is generally not attainable while operating unless you use a microscope or procedure scope. Naturally, it is impossible to maintain perfect posture at all times during procedures, and one postural guideline will not be comfortable for all body types. Therefore, it is helpful to know the recommended postural working ranges for each area of the body. (Fig. 3) Operators can use these guidelines to find a posture that best suits their body and then operate within these postural limits.

## Fig. 3: Recommended postural working ranges in dentistry

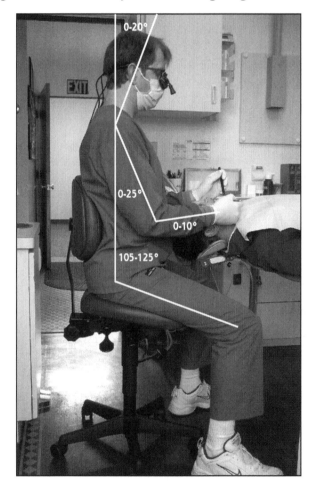

Using magnification, operators should strive for a head posture of no more then 20 degrees forward, the absolute maximum being 25 degrees.[13] The hip angle should be greater than 90 degrees to decrease pressure on the internal organs[11] and to help maintain the lumbar lordosis.[14] Recommended hip angles range from 105 degrees with a tilting seat pan to 125 degrees with a saddle stool. The thighs should be sloping downward, with the feet flat on the floor. However, operators with exaggerated curvature of the lumbar spine (hyperlordosis) may find that sitting on a sloping seat pan accentuates the lordosis and is uncomfortable.[15] You should feel weight evenly distributed three ways: through your buttocks and through each foot. Reaching forward from the shoulders up to 25 degrees and arm abduction up to 20 degrees are considered acceptable.[12] Forearms should be parallel to the floor or sloping about 10 degrees upward. Intermittently, when standing for injections or forceful extractions, 5 degrees to 10 degrees downward will provide greater leverage and enable slightly greater elbow torque production.[11]

Proper adjustment of the operator stool is imperative to attaining balanced seated posture. Use the guidelines on page 28 to attain a working posture that is within the aforementioned postural working range.

One anthropometric variable that can affect dental operator posture is *upper arm length*. Operators with short upper arms may find it easier to work with the oral cavity positioned at elbow height and forearms parallel to the floor. Those with longer upper arms may find it necessary to raise the patient slightly higher than the elbow so forearms are sloping very slightly upward. This will allow more freedom of leg movement around the patient headrest. It must be remembered that the further one deviates from "neutral" postures, the more force is exerted on muscles, joints and soft tissue.

Because is easy to lose the feeling of proper posture while working chairside, it is important to practice the following dental postural awareness exercise. (Fig. 4) This exercise not only reinforces proper neutral posture, but can also help correct accumulated postural muscle imbalances.

# Dental Postural Awareness Exercise

- Sit on a seat pan that is very slightly tilted forward or a saddle stool. Do not lean on the backrest throughout this exercise. Arch your back, then flatten it (or slouch). Alternate between these two

## ADJUSTING THE OPERATOR STOOL

To attain balanced seated posture, follow these adjustment steps:

- Adjust the backrest height so the most convex portion nestles in your low-back curve.
- Move the backrest away from your back.
- Sit all the way back on the seat.
- Tilt the seat slightly forward (up to 15 degrees)
- Adjust the height with feet flat on the floor so your thighs slope slightly downward. Your weight should be evenly distributed in a tripod pattern: each foot on the floor and your seat pan.

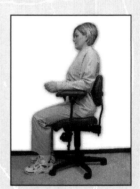

- Find your neutral pelvic position by alternately arching, then slouching the low back. Find a comfortable position between the two, and stabilize by pulling navel to spine. Hold this position.
- Bring the backrest forward to snugly contact the curve of your low back.
- Have someone else adjust your armrest height so your arms feel fully supported and relaxed, without visibly elevating the shoulders.

NOTE: If, at the highest adjustment, your thighs are parallel with the floor or only very slightly sloping downward, consider ordering a taller cylinder. On the other hand, if you cannot sit all the way back on the seat pan with your weight equally distributed through each foot and buttocks at the lowest adjustment, try a shorter cylinder. (Chapter 6)

extremes several times, then find a comfortable position in-between the two extremes.

- Hold this position by pulling your navel to your spine. Keep your navel pulled to spine throughout the exercise.
- Sit tall in your chair, lifting your chest toward the ceiling.

- Stretch your head toward the ceiling, as if there were a string attached to the back of your head pulling upward.

- Breathe in and point your thumbs backward, like a hitchhiker. (Fig. 4, left) Press shoulder blades down and together. Hold briefly.

- *Without letting your shoulders roll forward*, let your palms turn inward and relax at your sides while you slowly exhale. (Fig. 4, right)

- Hold the position for about one minute, then relax. Perform this exercise daily until this seated posture becomes a habit. (While operating, your head posture will probably be slightly forward. However the shoulders and trunk should maintain this balanced posture.)

- To develop optimal posture while standing, try this: After letting your palms return to your sides, stand up from the dental chair while holding this neutral posture. Then try walking with this neutral posture. This exercise should also be practiced outside the operatory to reinforce the feeling of neutral posture.

## Fig. 4: Dental postural awareness exercise

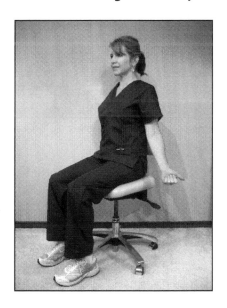 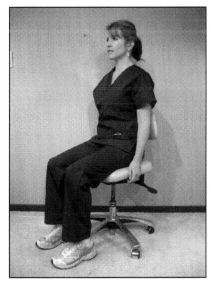

Maintaining this optimal operating posture whenever feasible is an effective tool to build and maintain optimal musculoskeletal health. As you will see, it must be considered in context of other factors involved, including not only proper equipment selection and adjustment, but also proper operator and patient positioning.

# Patient Positioning

After finding your neutral operating posture and adjusting your stool, position the patient. The quality of this positioning can greatly impact your posture. Remember that the patient is in the operatory room for only 45 to 60 minutes—you are there for your career. It's therefore imperative to take the time to position your patient strategically to accommodate your best working posture.

It has been shown that dentists who take the time to carefully position their patients to promote a direct view have significantly fewer headaches.[16] Optimal patient positioning requires several strategies: reclined angle of patient chair, proper chair and headrest adjustment, use of cervical positioning aids, verbal instructions to the patient, retracting aids, height adjustment and lighting.

General guidelines for patient positioning are to place the patient in supine for the maxillary treatment and semisupine for the mandibular treatment. These guidelines will vary depending on patient tolerance to supine, procedure type, location of treatment surface and other variables.[17] Inevitably there will be some patients who physically cannot be reclined properly due to postural hypotension, inner ear issues, vertigo and a myriad of other conditions. This means they must remain in a more upright position, placing the treatment area higher and more forward, making access difficult. These cases may best be treated with the operator standing or using a saddle stool to gain better proximity and view of the oral cavity. Remember, even when standing, to always perform the Operator Pivot when leaving neutral posture to protect and stabilize your back. (Chapter 3)

## *Recline the patient*

One of the most prevalent positioning problems I encounter is operators not reclining the backrest of the patient chair far enough. This promotes twisting, bending and leaning to view the oral cavity. Some patients are difficult to position due to their psychological inability to tolerate the supine position. To get these patients into a near-supine position, try these four "reclining" strategies:

- *Start low.* Before your patient arrives, recline the chair beyond the fully upright position. This way, when you recline the chair, it won't feel as dramatic to the patient.

- *Meet them halfway.* After your patient is seated, recline the chair back further than you actually desire. When your patient protests and insists upon sitting more upright, say "O.K., I'll meet you halfway." Now he or she is closer to your preferred position.

- *Doctor's orders.* For very problematic patients, have the dentist position the patient, if time permits. Patients may be less inclined to resist supine positioning from the doctor vs. an auxiliary.

- *Must-see TV.* Position a TV monitor, a hanging mobile or a picture on the ceiling, so the patient will be distracted while reclining.

# Headrest Positioning

With the patient properly reclined, (either semisupine or supine) the next objective is to position the patient's head to attain a more optimal view of the treatment area. Strategies will vary depending upon whether your patient chairs are equipped with a flat or a double articulating headrest.

## *Flat headrests*

Ask the patient to move all the way to the end of the headrest. Leaving "dead" space at the end of the headrest causes you to reach or lean forward and strains the back, neck and shoulder muscles.

This is especially important while treating at the 12 o'clock position. This repositioning towards you may cause some shorter patients to be uncomfortably out of alignment with the chair's natural lumbar support. This is easily resolved by placing lumbar, cervical and/or knee supports under the patient. (Fig. 5)

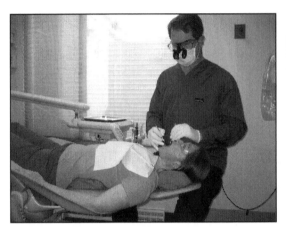

**Fig. 5: Proper patient positioning in a chair with flat headrest, using cervical and lumbar supports**

The flat headrest allows you to position the patient's head in three axes: tilting the head up or down, rotating the head and side-bending the head to the side. (Fig. 6) Tilt the patient's head to the desired degree using a cervical roll or pillow behind the neck. You may also try a wedge cushion under the upper part of the patient's back, which has been shown to significantly reduce dentist's musculoskeletal complaints.[18] Positioning with ergonomic cushions can also greatly improve your patient's comfort. Neck rotation can be achieved with verbal cues, and side-bending the head to one side is best achieved manually.

Geriatric patients frequently have exaggerated (kyphotic) forward head posture. These patients are more comfortable when supported with a double articulating headrest angled forward, or a large soft pillow behind the neck to support the head in a forward posture. Since this positioning keeps the head forward and can make access difficult, it is important to recline the chair of geriatric patients as far as possible. These patients can often be more comfortably treated when the operator is standing or halfway between standing and sitting (i.e., using a saddle-style stool).

**Fig. 6: The flat headrest allows positioning of the patient's head in three axes: tilting up or down, side-bending, and rotation.**

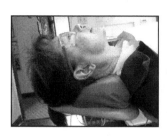 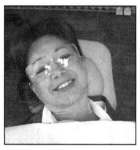 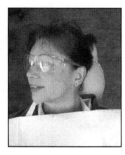

## *Double articulating headrests*

The head can be positioned in two axes with a double articulating headrest: tilting up or down and rotation. For maxillary procedures with nongeriatric patients, angle the headrest up into the occiput, which will help relax the patient's neck muscles, position the chin higher and enable better viewing of the oral cavity. (Fig. 7, left)

Since length of double articulating headrests varies with manufacturer, be sure the patient moves all the way to the end of the headrest. For mandibular procedures, keep the headrest flatter (you may still want to use a neck support) and move it slightly forward. (Fig. 7, right)

**Fig. 7: Patient positioning for maxillary and mandibular procedures**

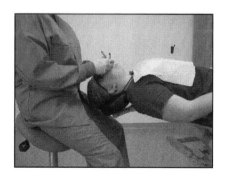 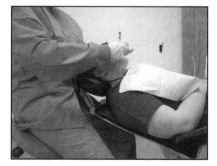

## Proper height

Next, position the patient at the proper height to accommodate your balanced operating posture. The height of the patient should enable you to operate within the recommended postural working range for all areas of the body. (Fig. 3) A good guideline for achieving proper height is to position the working surface (occlusal surface) at elbow level or slightly higher while operating.[12] Placing the patient too high is a common mistake that can cause shoulder elevation or arm abduction (especially in the 8 o'clock to 10 o'clock positions)—both risk factors for neck and shoulder pain.

## Friendly reminders

Ask the patient to turn his or her head for easy access. As the patient's head inevitably drifts away from you, continue the verbal cues to keep the head turned. Position the patient appropriately for the quadrant to be treated and to enable a line of sight that is perpendicular to the occlusal surface. For example, during treatment of the lower right quadrant (buccal side) you will want the patient's head turned toward the assistant.[17] Remember, the patient's head also bends to the side. So if you have a flat headrest, try side-bending the patient's head toward you and *then* ask them to turn their head for select procedures. This can often help position the oral cavity two inches to three inches closer to you and enable enhanced viewing of the treatment area.[19]

## Equipment placement

Position your delivery system and any other frequently used dental instruments or equipment within easy fingertip reach. Equipment used less frequently can be placed farther away or placed on a mobile cart for use in multiple rooms.

## See the light

The operatory light should be adjusted to minimize the need to leave a neutral working posture. Traditional schools of thought on lighting positions have recommended placing the light directly over the oral cavity for the mandibular arch and angled up over the chest of the patient for the maxillary arch. Unfortunately, it is easy to get shadowing with the latter method of illumination.[20] To prevent shadowing, the light should be aimed perpendicularly onto the occlusal surface. An alternate lighting method is to position the operatory light parallel to (or within 15 degrees of) the operator's *line of sight.* This will usually require the light to be located slightly behind the operator's head for the lower arch in the 11 o'clock to 12 o'clock positions.[20] For the upper arch, a mirror may be used to reflect light onto the surface.

Use of a headlight mounted to operating scopes or on a headband places light directly upon the area being viewed. This reduces or eliminates shadows, increases visual acuity and decreases the need for operator or assistant to constantly reposition the operatory light. In fact, overhead lights can sometimes be nearly eliminated with this direct illumination.

# Operator Positioning

There is ongoing debate regarding optimal operator position in modern dental practice. From dentists who operate exclusively in the 12 o'clock position to hygienists who side-sit at the 8 o'clock position, favored positions and their justifications vary widely.

Two primary goals in operator positioning are: To maintain an operating posture of the spine, neck, shoulder and wrist that is as close to neutral as possible (Fig. 3); and to develop comfortable seating in multiple positions around the patient's head to allow for movement and frequent change of positions. Obviously, operating exclusively in either of the above positions does not meet these goals. In Chapters 3 through 5, we will focus on how specific operator positions affect certain areas of the body. Here, I will describe some basics of operator positioning.

## *Location, location, location*

After properly positioning the patient and your equipment, determine which clock position (Fig. 8) provides a line of sight that is perpendicular to the working surface (direct or indirect vision) and preserves your optimal working posture. For example, while treating the occlusal surface of tooth no. 3 (sealant or direct restoration), an indirect view at 11 o'clock to 12 o'clock positions would enable a perpendicular line of sight. On the other hand, the lingual surface of tooth no. 19 may be better seen from the 9 o'clock to 10 o'clock positions with a direct view.[17] Recommendations for operator and assistant positioning for specific tooth surfaces is beyond the scope of this book and available in the "Resources" section.

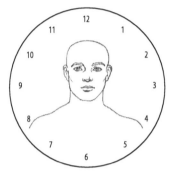

**Fig. 8: Operator positions in relation to the patient are described in terms of "clock" positions**

In general, the 11 o'clock to 1 o'clock positions enable some of the most neutral operator postures, especially of the arms, and should be made easily accessible in the operatory.[21] Frequent positioning at the 10 o'clock position without a mirror tends to encourage more arm abduction and neck/shoulder problems.[18,21] With all positions, use of indirect vision using the mirror is an important ergonomic consideration to maintain neutral postures.

## *Tools of the trade*

Indirect vision utilizing a mirror will enable the best operator posture for some areas of the mouth (for example, occlusal surfaces of the upper arch). Mirrors should be used whenever direct viewing of the oral cavity requires leaving neutral posture. One study revealed that more pain-free dentists use a mirror in the 10 o'clock position than those who did not utilize a mirror.[18] While this seems self-evident, I have observed many operators with pain issues unnecessarily contort their bodies to visualize the treatment area instead of using the mirror.

Retraction of soft tissue with positioning aids can alleviate the need for sustained, manual retraction and may help prevent pain syndromes in the left (mirror or retracting-side) arm and shoulder. Use a rubber dam or cheek retractors to minimize manual retracting of these areas. (Chapter 6)

## *Change positions frequently*

Since prolonged, static postures are a primary cause of CTDs in dentistry, try to change positions frequently around the head of the patient.[22] Every time you move, you subtly shift the workload from one group of muscles to another. This decreases the chances of over-working one group of muscles and also of developing muscle ischemia. Try to spend slightly more time in the 11 o'clock to 1 o'clock positions and less in the 8 o'clock to 10 o'clock positions, especially if you have a patient chair with wide "wings," which requires leaning forward and inhibits close positioning.

For some procedures, dentists may find that standing affords them a better ergonomic position than sitting. (Chapter 3)

## SEQUENCE FOR POSITIONING SUCCESS

1. **Operator posture.** Always establish proper operator posture first. This includes neutral posture exercise, proper chair adjustment, height, seat tilt and armrest adjustment (optional).

2. **Patient position.** Adjust the patient to accommodate your neutral posture. This process involves:

   - Degree of reclining (supine vs. semisupine)
   - Moving patient to end of headrest
   - Adjusting the head tilt appropriately for desired arch
   - Patient chair height
   - Head position: rotation and/or head side-bending (if using a flat headrest)
   - Positioning equipment within easy reach
   - Adjusting light to prevent shadowing

3. **Operator position.** Move to the appropriate clock position to preserve your neutral posture.

   - Establish a direct line of view that is perpendicular to the occlusal surface. This may be direct or indirect, depending upon the quadrant.
   - Change positions as frequently as possible.

## Don't side-sit

Side-sitting at the 9 o'clock position requires twisting the torso and places the hip, shoulder and neck in non-neutral postures.[11] (Fig. 9) Holding this unbalanced posture for prolonged periods of time can cause adaptive muscle shortening[1] and put you on the fast-track to low back and shoulder problems. If positioning at 9 o'clock is difficult due to a patient chair with wide "wings," consider using a saddle stool to gain closer proximity by opening the hip angle. (Fig. 10)

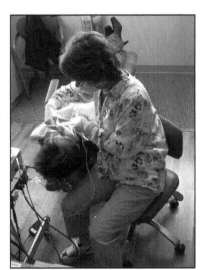

**Fig. 9: Side-sitting at the 9 o'clock position can lead to a myriad of musculoskeletal problems**

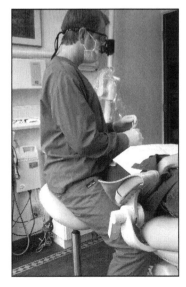

**Fig. 10: A saddle stool can help maintain proper posture at the 9 o'clock position by opening the hip angle**

# Periodic Stretching

Your life is busy. You have 25 hours worth of work to do in a 24-hour day. But it's important to take frequent breaks during the day to stretch and move. Incorporating regular breaks for chairside stretching and movement into your workday can put you on the path toward a longer and healthier career.[16,20,23,24]

Studies show that dentists' pain complaints have risen since the 1960s due, in part, to longer work periods without breaks.[25,26] As described in Chapter 1, these prolonged static postures (PSPs) cause significant microtrauma in your body that can lead to work-related pain and CTDs in dentistry.

Chairside stretching is a strategy that addresses nearly every microtrauma resulting from PSPs.

Stretching helps *prevent muscle imbalances* by maintaining normal range of motion and improving flexibility.[27,28] When assuming awkward PSPs during treatment, you become predisposed to developing muscle imbalances. This is because operators tend to repeatedly flex forward, bend to the side and rotate in one direction. In general, you tend to lose flexibility in directions opposite to those in which you are postured statically during the day.[18] Stretches performed in the reverse direction of awkward prolonged, static postures improves flexibility and helps prevent muscle imbalances that can lead to pain and CTDs.

Chairside stretching also:
- *Prevents muscle ischemia* by increasing blood flow to muscles. Even in perfect neutral working posture, more than half of your body's muscles are working. Static muscle contractions can cause ischemia.[29] Dynamic movement into and out of stretches provides nourishment for your muscles. It increases blood flow, oxygen and nutrients to your muscles and "warms" them up.[30]
- *Reduces formation of painful trigger points.* Prolonged static postures cause stiff, underused, tight muscles that are prone to developing ischemia and trigger points. The mechanism of gentle stretching helps treat and prevent trigger points.[31] Stretching also is extremely relaxing, an important consideration since emotional stress spawns trigger points.[31]

- *Prevents disc degeneration* by increasing nutrient supply to the disc. After about age 30, your spinal discs no longer receive nutrients via bloodflow.[6] An important way the disc receives nutrients is by movement—alternately compressing and releasing the disc pressure. When the disc releases, it absorbs nutrients.[6] Therefore, stretching helps the discs absorb water and nutrients and remain healthy.

Stretches can be performed in or out of the operatory and should be incorporated into a daily routine. Chairside stretching involves a rotation, side-bending or extension component that generally is in the opposite direction of that in which you commonly work.

## *Microbreaks*

In professional sports, athletes are admired for toughing-out injuries. That may be appropriate for people whose careers often span less than a decade. For dentists, it can be a career-killer. This is why frequent short breaks (microbreaks) are important. Stretching, rest or movement can be performed during microbreaks to allow repair of microtrauma. In fact, a study on the efficacy of microbreaks during the workday found that people who regularly scheduled microbreaks experienced less discomfort and showed no detrimental effect on productivity.[32] Another study found that dentists who utilized naturally occurring breaks during their workday to rest or move had significantly less pain and discomfort.[18] Other authors have also pointed to the efficacy of using micropauses and stretching during dental procedures.[20,23,24] The most recent study on the effects of stretching revealed that static stretching can improve other aspects of exercise performance, especially strength and endurance.[33]

If these breaks are too far apart, the rate of damage will exceed the rate of repair, ultimately resulting in breakdown of tissue. To optimize your strength capacity and minimize the risk of muscle strain, a schedule of brief, frequent rest periods is more beneficial than lengthy infrequent rest periods.[11]

The duration of the stretch you perform during a microbreak is also important. A sustained 15- or 30-second stretch has been shown to be more effective than brief, repeated five-second stretches (a.k.a. DROM stretching).[27,28] You may perform a chairside stretch lasting 15 seconds (two to three breathing cycles) every 30 minutes to 45 minutes. At home, you may hold stretches for 20 seconds to 30 seconds, or longer.

The stretches introduced in this book have been designed to be easily performed chairside while wearing gloves and without cross contamination. There are countless times during the workday when you and your staff can squeeze in a microbreak. Some examples include:

### Dentists

- While assistant is light curing
- While assistant is making alginate impressions
- Waiting for anesthesia
- During failed appointments or between patients

### Hygienists

- Breaks during educational patient videos
- During a fluoride treatment
- Waiting for anesthesia
- Before reaching for instruments

### Assistants

- While dentist is sculpting a composite or carving an amalgam
- While dentist consults with patient on procedure
- During dentist recall exam
- During impression-making by dentist

Chairside stretches should also be performed outside the operatory—use your imagination. You can also benefit simply by standing up during a break, taking a short walk or performing other activities involving movement during longer breaks or at lunch.

## How to stretch safely

It is imperative to learn to stretch properly. An improperly performed stretch can actually promote injuries. First, assume the starting position for the stretch, breathe in deeply and exhale as you slowly increase the intensity of the stretch up to a point of mild tension or discomfort. Hold the stretch for two to three breathing cycles, then slowly release the stretch and return to a neutral position. Repeat the stretch, as time allows. Perform stretches in both directions, to determine if one side is tighter than the other. If bilateral tightness is present, perform the stretch primarily toward the tightest side throughout the workday. At home, perform stretches in both directions. Avoid stretching in a painful range, and discontinue stretching if it increases pain. The same stretch may be performed up to three times daily—more, if advised by a healthcare professional.

## Selection of stretches

A chairside stretching program for dentists and hygienists should help prevent unique pain syndromes and imbalances to which dental professionals are predisposed. Naturally, you will not want to target and stretch muscles that are prone to weakness and lengthening, so you should be prudent with your selection of stretches. Stretches should be easy to perform chairside *with* gloves on and reverse common unbalanced operating postures. While several stretches on the following chart are common "staples" in the physical therapy profession, others were developed specifically for the dental profession by the author. For example, the "Un-twister" stretch was developed by the author based on a Swedish dental study revealing a limited range of motion among dentists,[34] and a Japanese dental study that demonstrated repeated asymmetrical posturing.[35]

For optimal benefit, it is a good idea to observe and refresh proper stretching techniques either in an educational environment or via video. It is also helpful to hang stretching wall charts in the operatory or staff lounge. Dental chairside stretching DVDs and laminated stretching wall charts are available at *www.posturedontics.com*. Regular stretching, both chairside and out of the operatory, is an important lifestyle adjustment that can put you on the path toward a longer and healthier career.

## Fig. 11: Examples of chairside stretches for dental professionals

(From *Smart Moves for Dental Professionals in the Operatory;
Chairside Stretching* DVD. Available at www.posturedontics.com.)

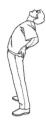

**The Reversal**

Support wrists on hips
and slowly lean backward.
Do not over-extend
the head. Hold for 2-4
breath cycles.

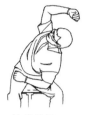

**The Un-Twister**

Legs in tripod position, bend to your
left side, resting left elbow on left knee.
Stretch right arm overhead and look
toward ceiling. Hold for 2-4 breath
cycles.

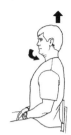

**The Chin Nod**

Strengthens postural neck muscles.
Lift chest upward, shoulders back.
Nod the head, dipping the chin
slightly downward. Hold 1 slow
breath cycle. Repeat 5 times.

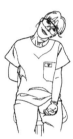

**Scalene Stretch
(Ear-to-Shoulder)**

Anchor right hand behind your back
or chair. Slowly bring left ear toward
left shoulder. Hold 2-4 breath cycles.

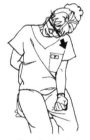

**Trapezius Stretch
(Ear-to-Armpit)**

Anchor right hand behind your back
or chair. Slowly bring left ear toward
left armpit. Hold 2-4 breath cycles.

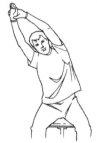

**Overhead Stretch**

Sit tall, clasp hands over head with
palms toward ceiling. Bend trunk to
one side. Hold for 2-4 breath cycles.

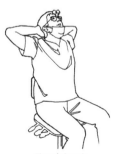

**Thoracic Stretch**

Clasp fingers together behind
occiput and slowly extend the upper
back. Look toward ceiling and press
the elbows outward to stretch the
chest.

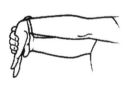

**Wrist Extensor Stretch**

With straight elbow, point fingers
downward and gently pull fingers
and hand toward the body.
Hold 2-4 breath cycles.

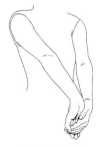

**Carpal Tunnel Stretch**

Turn the palm upward and hold the
palm as you slowly extend the elbow
until straight. Hold 2-4 breath
cycles.

***Disclaimer:*** *The sample stretches presented are for persons who are in good general health. If you have been injured, suffer from a medical condition or are under a medical professional's care, consult with a licensed medical practitioner before beginning these stretches. Not all stretches are suitable for everyone. As with any exercise, improper performance or overuse may lead to pain or worsening of symptoms. (For more information on Red Flag precautions and exercise guidelines, see Chapters 8 and 9 or consult your physician.)*

CHAPTER THREE

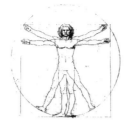

# Why Let Plaque
# Be a Pain in the Back?

Though no one can go back and make a brand new start,
anyone can start from now and make a brand new ending.

CARL BARD

Chances are good that you have experienced low-back pain at some point in your life. More than three out of four adults in the United States experience back pain at some point in their lives.[1] In a given year, between 10 percent and 17 percent of adults in the United States experience low-back pain;[2] however, among U.S. dentists and hygienists, the prevalence of low-back pain is 37 percent to 63 percent.[3-6] Low-back pain is a primary cause of occupational disability and costs the U.S. economy $90 billion annually.[7]

Two of the primary contributing factors to low-back pain among dental professionals are static, poor seated postures and muscle imbalances due to weak stabilizing muscles of the trunk. Since operator seating has a direct impact on low-back posture, we will begin with seated operator posture.

45

# Seated Low-Back Posture

A reclined, seated posture places the least amount of stress on the low back discs and muscles.[8] Of course, it's impossible to practice dentistry in a reclined position.

Attaining a healthy seated working posture can be surprisingly difficult for many dentists and their staff, and it can dramatically impact low-back pain. It's not at all uncommon to see operators slouching, perched on the edge of their stools or in other unhealthy working postures.

Let's examine some common seated postures, how they occur in the operatory, and how they affect your low-back health.

| Fig. 1A | Fig. 1B | Fig. 1C | Fig. 1D |
|---|---|---|---|
| Pelvis is rolled backward in passive sitting on a flat seat causing flattening of the low-back curve. | Pelvis is held in a neutral position through active sitting on a flat seat, requiring constant contraction of back muscles, which quickly fatigues them. | Pelvis is more balanced with less muscular effort on a tilted seat pan or saddle stool, minimizing the need for backrest support. | Pelvis is rolled forward when too much seat tilt is used or from congenital abnormality causing excessive lordosis, or swayback posture. |

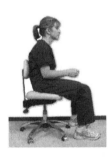 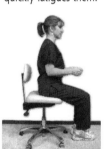 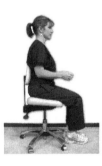 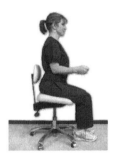

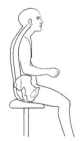 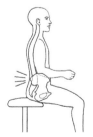 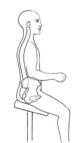 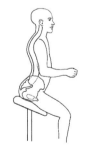

## Passive sitting

Passive sitting, which looks like slouching, is a common posture in the operatory because it expends very little energy. On a flat seatpan, the pelvis rolls backward (Fig. 1A), causing the lumbar curve to flatten. Since nearly every curve of the spine affects the curve above or below it, the flattened low-back curve causes a reciprocal forward movement of the head. In this C-shaped posture, the operator's spine is providing little support, and the body is literally hanging on the soft structures at the back of the spine. The flattened lumbar curve significantly increases the load on muscles and spinal discs.[9] It also can stretch and permanently elongate the iliolumbar ligaments (a.k.a., "creep"), decreasing spinal stability.[7,10]

Over time, ligaments, muscles and soft tissue may stretch or shorten to adapt to a slouched working posture and hold the spine in unbalanced posture. Muscle strains, headaches and trigger points, as well as possible disc degeneration or herniation result from this posturing.[11]

## Active sitting

Remember your mother always telling you to sit up straight? You also may have heard a version of this in dental or hygiene school, or even at an ergonomics seminar. While it is obvious that good posture is key to injury prevention in dentistry, this advice is often given without context or specific instructions. Commanding operators to "sit up straight" encourages most of them to assume active sitting. (Fig. 1B)

Although the pelvis tends to roll backward on a flat seat pan, the pelvis may be actively forced into a more neutral position through constant contraction of the back extensor muscles, which help maintain your lumbar curve.[12] Unfortunately, this posture places greater loads on the spine than does standing, uses up significant energy, and cannot be maintained for very long.[8,13] When your muscles finally fatigue, you simply slump into passive sitting. A backrest can help reduce muscle fatigue and promote a neutral posture; however, while operating, you are usually leaning on the backrest less than half of the time.

Learning how to properly "sit up straight" involves correct use of the transverse abdominal muscles (those are the abs that run horizontally around your midsection, similar to a corset), proper chair adjustment, seat selection, specific endurance training of certain back muscles—the erector spinae (large muscles on either side of your spine) and multifidus muscles (small muscles located close to your spine, deep in your low back)—and proper working distance and declination angle of your scopes. (Fig. 1C)

This is a lot of information to absorb. Try to think of each part of your body as a tool with a specific function (which it is). You wouldn't use a hammer to install a screw, so why would you force the structures of your back to assume postures it wasn't meant to hold? This is why it's crucial to find a seating option that places the pelvis in its most neutral position so it balances the spine, reduces muscle strain and decreases disc pressure.[14] As we will see, spinal disc degeneration and herniation are directly impacted by low-back posture.

# Spinal Discs and Degeneration

Located between your spinal vertebrae are spinal discs which allow movement of the spine. Inside each disc is the gel-like nucleus which functions similar to a water balloon. Vertical forces cause the nucleus to deform and flatten. When the force decreases, the nucleus returns to its normal shape. The occupation of dentistry puts the operator at risk for injuring the disc in three primary ways.

First, prolonged, static postures reduce nutrition to discs and nuclei. Since there is no blood supply to the inside of the disc, its only means of nutrition is via imbibition.[11] Think of the disc as a sponge. At rest, it absorbs no water; however, when compressed and released, it imbibes water. This is similar to the mechanism of the spinal disc. (Fig. 2) It requires alternate compression and relaxation to stay healthy. Therefore, movement is essential to the health of your spinal discs.

Next, sustained contractions in the muscles that extend your spine (as during active sitting) also reduce disc nutrition by compressing the discs, increasing intra-discal pressure.[15]

## Fig. 2: Spinal disc and nucleus gain nutrition through alternate compression and release

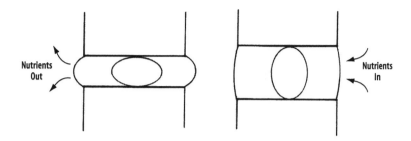

Nutrients Out

Nutrients In

Finally, lumbar disc pressures are generally higher in sitting than in standing. When you are not in contact with a lumbar support (as occurs frequently in dentistry) the disc pressure rises dramatically. Compared to a neutral standing posture, lumbar disc pressures increase by 40 percent when you sit "actively" (without leaning on a backrest), and by 200 percent when sitting and leaning forward 40 degrees.[16] This has particular relevance to dentistry since studies show that dentists and hygienists tend to lean forward at least 30 degrees for more than half of their working hours.[17] Incidentally, lumbar disc loads always decrease when the back is in contact with a lumbar support.[8]

# Herniated Discs and End-Plate Fractures

If you've felt stabbing low-back pain or shooting pain into your hind quarters or down the back of your leg, you might think you've suddenly damaged the area. This is usually incorrect. A structural problem has probably existed for a while; you just didn't notice it. A common cause of this type of neuropathy is a spinal disc herniation or end-plate fracture.

For true disc herniation to occur, typically the spine must be bent forward repeatedly.[18] Considering that dentists and hygienists lean their trunks forward over half of their operating hours,[17] the possibility of this mechanism as an etiology is quite likely. The frequency of this type of injury also is highest in sedentary seated occupations and is more common in younger spines than in older ones.[18]

When bending forward, the nucleus of the spinal disc pushes against the posterior wall of the spinal disc. (Fig. 3) Over time, repeated forward bending can cause weakening and wearing away of the disc layers from the inside out. In the early stages, you may not feel much, since the inner disc wall has no nerves.[12] At this point, your condition is still reversible. Two-thirds of your spinal disc can be damaged or worn away before you ever feel pain. (This is why many dentists report episodes of herniated or bulging discs as happening "suddenly, or without warning.") There's actually nothing sudden about it. After years of spinal disc microtrauma, the weakened disc wall can bulge backward, putting pressure on the spinal cord or peripheral nerves, causing low back, hip or leg pain, numbness or tingling.

This is where the shooting pain can develop, and it's time to schedule a session with a physical therapist. If you ignore the pain, your problem can worsen easily. The nucleus could actually extrude from the disc (herniation). That means surgery—or, possibly, the end of your career.

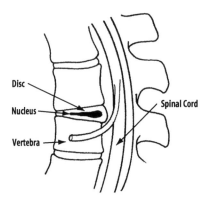

Disc
Nucleus
Spinal Cord
Vertebra

**Fig. 3: A common theory for low-back pain: flattening of the lumbar curve, which causes the nucleus to weaken the disc wall, can lead to a bulging or herniated disc**

More current research finds that end-plate vertebral fractures are a common and frequently misdiagnosed etiology, resulting in the same nerve compression and symptoms as a herniated disc.[18] In this scenario, the fluid of the nucleus is squeezed (upward, for example) through a crack in the endplate of an adjacent vertebra, into the vertebral bone due to compressive loading of the nucleus. Researchers have found that an audible "pop" occurs with this mechanism, similar to what patients who have a diagnosis of disc herniation report. To stay healthy, the nucleus must stay centered inside the spinal disc when standing and sitting, which requires a neutral posture. Spinal discs also require movement to stay healthy, so prolonged, static muscle contractions must be minimized. Finally, high compressive disc loads can weaken end-plates, so proper seating, exercise and weight loads must be selected.

# Muscle Imbalances

Imbalances that develop between your abdominal and low-back muscles are especially problematic in seated dentistry. Repeatedly leaning toward a patient can cause strain and overexertion in the superficial back extensor muscles, while the deep stabilizing trunk muscles (transverse and oblique abdominals, quadratus lumborum, multifidus) tend to become weaker.

Two 1996 studies demonstrated the importance of proper strength and control of the deepest abdominal muscle, the transverse abdominal muscle, in the prevention of low-back pain.[19,20] Another study showed that only 10 percent of patients with a history of low-back pain could effectively contract the transverse abdominal muscle, compared with 82 percent of non-symptomatic subjects. The ability to effectively contract this muscle was closely linked to patients' reports of decreased pain levels, expressions that the back felt safer and their ability to control back pain.[21]

## UPPER BACK PAIN

Though not as common as low-back pain, upper-back pain may be experienced among team members. The thoracic spine attaches to the ribs, forming a rigid encasement that protects the lungs and vital organs. It is less mobile than the cervical and lumbar spine, so trauma here is rarely due to disc degeneration. More often, this type of pain is from muscles and ligaments.[36] Referred pain from trigger points easily develop in the thoracic paraspinal muscles and rhomboids due to stooped postures and sustained reaching in front of the body, as is common in dentistry.[37] Trigger point treatment is described in Chapter 8.

More recent research by McGill demonstrates the importance of strength and proper abdominal bracing using all *three* abdominal wall layers, including external, internal and transverse abdominals to stabilize the spine. Utilization of all three muscle groups may actually be a more effective means of protecting the low back than recruitment of the transverse abdominal muscle alone.[18]

Another problematic muscle imbalance affecting the low back is caused by the tendency of right-handed dentists to lean forward and to the right for two-thirds of their operating hours. Compared to other dentists in the study, these dentists had the highest incidence of neck, back and shoulder pain.[22] Prolonged, forward and side leaning can lead to adaptive muscle shortening (Chapter 1) in the low back musculature. This unbalanced posture has been shown to be the primary posture contributing to disc bulge and herniation.[9]

# Joint Mobility

Operators who repeatedly lean forward toward patients may have excellent or excessive spinal flexion; but, over time, the ability of the spine to extend is diminished. The loss of mobility can lead to early degenerative changes in the joint and put the operator at risk for further injury.[23]

# Keys to Success: Preventing Low-Back Pain

Painful warning signs often alert us to damaging microtrauma. However, in the low-back, disc herniations can occur with little or no warning signs. It is therefore of paramount importance, when speaking of back pain, to practice prevention and implement conservative measures *before* painful episodes occur.

## *Neutral posture*

Maintaining neutral low-back posture in dentistry is essential in the prevention of low-back pain and your career longevity in dentistry. This means maintaining a slight curve in the low back when seated or standing.

In dental or hygiene school, you were probably taught to sit with your thighs parallel to the floor, or your hips at a 90-degree angle on a flat seat pan. This seating encourages the pelvis to roll backward and flatten the low-back curve. (Fig. 1A)[2,9,24] Your only options to maintain your lumbar curve on a flat seat pan are to either maintain constant contact with a well-designed lumbar support or sit actively. Maintaining constant, snug contact with a backrest is nearly impossible in dentistry due to the inevitable need to intermittently lean forward to view the oral cavity, and active sitting, as discussed earlier, requires constant contraction of the back muscles and can usually be maintained for only short periods of time.

In dentistry, an easier method to maintain your neutral pelvic position, which facilitates your natural low back curve, involves the use of a seat pan tilted slightly forward[25] (Fig. 1C) and adjusting the stool height so your hips are positioned slightly higher than your knees.[8,26] This rotates your pelvis forward to a more neutral position, (as in standing), brings more balance to the curves of your spine and facilitates more dynamic body movement. Maintaining this curve reduces disc pressure, helping reduce low-back pain,[27] and the downward slope of the thighs usually enables closer positioning to the patient.

**Fig. 4: A saddle stool places the pelvis in a near-neutral position, which balances the spinal curves and minimizes muscle strain.**

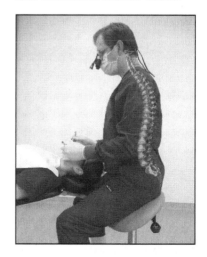

Sitting with the seat pan tilted forward 5 degrees to 15 degrees opens the hip angle to about 110 degrees, while a saddle-style stool increases the angle to about 125 degrees or more. Using a saddle stool (Fig. 4) moves your pelvis toward its most neutral seated position (very close to a standing posture), which requires the least muscular effort to

## TALL OPERATORS

One of the most common problems I see among tall dentists with low-back pain is sitting too low, which causes flattening of the lumbar curve. Make sure that at the highest chair adjustment, you are not sitting with your thighs parallel to the floor, or worse, knees higher than hips. Sitting higher helps maintain your natural low back curve and, when the back is unsupported, decreases low back muscle activity.[38] You may need to order a tall stool cylinder (a tall "lift") from your dental manufacturer to retrofit your too-low seat. A saddle stool also can be helpful for taller operators to sit higher. Remember that whenever dentists change their operating height, this will affect the assistant, who must also change their position. Oftentimes, this provides a good opportunity for assistants to stand during treatment.

maintain the spinal curves. This is one reason the saddle stool does not usually require a backrest. Since these stools place compression on the peritoneal structures, comfort will vary between different designs and operators.

Tilting the seat pan too far forward (beyond 15 degrees) may cause the operator to slide forward on the seat pan, losing contact with the lumbar support, and may cause an excessive curve of the low back. (Fig. 1D) Individuals with hyperlordosis (extreme curvature of the low back) or spondylolisthesis may benefit less from a tilting seat pan, as it will further promote this curvature and may cause discomfort. Individuals with these postural dysfunctions should consult with an ergonomic specialist or healthcare professional to determine what seating is best for them.

Although difficult to utilize effectively in dentistry, the lumbar support is a key feature that has been shown to significantly reduce low-back pain by facilitating a lumbar lordosis and reducing muscle activity when used continuously.[8,28] Although dental operators cannot generally maintain constant contact with these supports throughout procedures, they are helpful to periodically allow relaxation of the lumbar musculature. These must be the proper size, shape and position to be effective. (Chapter 6)

Nontilting operator stools may be retrofitted with a wedge-shaped ergonomic cushion to economically gain the benefits of a tilting seat pan. (Fig. 5)

### Strengthen postural stabilizing muscles

The transverse abdominal, oblique abdominal, quadratus lumborum (which "hike" the hip on one side), and other key muscles play an important role in stabilizing the low back and maintaining the low back curve.[18,19] In addition to targeting these muscles in a strengthening

**Fig. 5: Nontilting seat pans may be retrofitted with an ergonomic seat cushion**

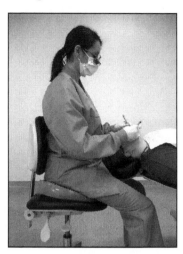

program (Chapter 9), dentists can regularly recruit them in the operatory to stabilize the back and prevent low-back pain.

In dentistry, you inevitably lean forward from time to time to gain better viewing of the oral cavity. When you do lean forward, extreme torque is placed on your back muscles and spinal discs. By stabilizing from the "inside out," with your transverse abdominal muscles, you dramatically decrease the stress on these muscles and spinal discs. Anytime your back is not supported on the back rest, these muscles should be recruited to protect, stabilize and maintain the low-back curve. This is done by performing the Dental Operator Pivot whenever you must lean forward to gain better visibility.

# Dental Operator Pivot Exercise

- Sit tall on the stool with a slight curve in the low back. (Fig. 6, left)

- Assume an operating position with the arms.

- To activate the transverse abdominal muscle, exhale, and actively (with your muscles) pull your navel toward your spine. (One common mistake is to suck in one's breath to pull the spine toward the navel. You should still be able to talk, breathe and move while holding this contraction.) An alternate method which utilizes all three abdominal wall layers is to 'brace' with the abdominal muscles, as though preparing for someone to hit you in the stomach.[18]

• Using the hips as a fulcrum, pivot forward from the hips, maintaining the abdominal contraction throughout the exercise. (Fig. 6, right)

Your abdominal muscles are now helping stabilize your low-back and are strengthened each time this exercise is performed. When standing, you should also use the operator pivot exercise to protect your low back when leaving a balanced, neutral posture.

**Fig. 6: The dental operator pivot exercise helps protect and stabilize the low back when leaving neutral operating postures**

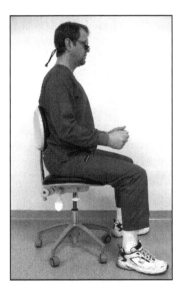 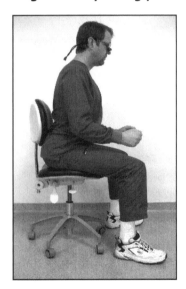

## *Work around the 'clock'*

A significant contributing factor to lower back pain and disc degeneration is staying in one seated working position.[18] Even very low-level static contractions (2 percent of maximum) of the low-back muscles cause oxygen deprivation when held for prolonged periods of time,[29] which can result in low-back pain. Regularly repositioning (8 o'clock to 1 o'clock) around the head of the patient shifts muscle workload from one area to another, preventing fatigue. If access behind the patient (11 o'clock to 1 o'clock positions) is restricted, try swiveling the patient chair about 20 degrees to gain access.

## *Switch up*

Sitting is not always better than standing. The low-back curve when standing is 50 percent greater than when sitting[30], and standing uses different muscle groups than sitting.[31] Therefore, alternating between the two positions allows for a dynamic working environment; one group of muscles rest while the workload is shifted to another muscle group.[25]

One study revealed that dentists who worked solely in a seated position had more severe low-back pain than did those who alternated between standing and sitting.[32] Dentists spend more than three-fourths of their total working hours seated. Hygienists may spend slightly less time seated if they clean their own rooms and equipment between patients. This may partially account for the higher incidence of low-back pain among dentists than hygienists. Operators should consider standing for treatment of the lower arch, geriatric patients, obese or large-chested patients and patients who cannot recline fully. In addition, dentists may stand for exams, extractions, removable prosthetic procedures and impression-making. Hygienists should consider standing when polishing and during fluoride treatments. Use your imagination to find times to stand regularly throughout your workday. (Fig. 7)

Research suggests that although sitting with hips higher than knees has many benefits, operators should still change spinal postures frequently.[18] Consider this strategy: alternate between a traditional operator chair with armrests and a saddle-style stool during the workday since each uses different muscle groups.

**Fig. 7: Standing reduces strain on lumbar spinal discs and may, for select procedures, enable a better ergonomic position than sitting**

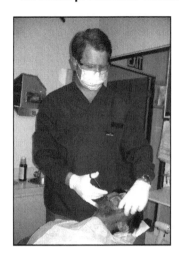 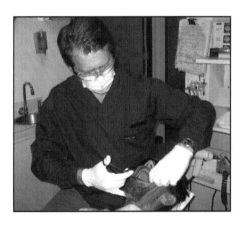

## *Avoid repeated twisting to one side*

Operatory design plays an important role in how often dentists perform detrimental twisting movements during the workday. Rear-delivery systems encourage extensive trunk twisting; side-delivery systems require moderate twisting; while continental, or over-the-patient, delivery systems minimize these movements. If the operatory design requires the dentist to turn to retrieve instruments or handpieces, the dentist should swivel the chair to face the area squarely instead of twisting the torso. Operators should try to retrieve items with the closest hand (especially with rear-delivery systems) to avoid twisting or reaching across the body. Repeated twisting in one direction may result in muscle imbalances or structural tissue damage, leading to low-back pain.[33,34]

## *Close proximity to the patient*

The farther the workload is from the spine, the more strain is produced on the trunk muscles and spinal discs,[12] so a very important concept in preventing back pain is to work close to the patient.[2] This can be challenging when working with poor ergonomic equipment: patient chairs with thick backs, wide upper backrests, knobs behind the patient headrest. A saddle stool in these situations can be helpful in getting closer to the patient.

Proximity may be a problem for many female dentists and hygienists due to physical barriers (large breasts, pregnancy) or modesty. If close positioning is difficult or impossible due to physical constraints, then armrests, specific exercises or postural bracing/support may be necessary. On the other hand, if operator modesty is preventing close proximity, the female operator must realize that musculoskeletal pain is a frequent trade-off for this modesty.

## *Periodic stretching/movement*

Staying flexible is an integral part of controlling low-back pain among dental professionals, especially men. Specific self-stretching exercises are one of the best preventive strategies for low-back pain.[11] Unilateral tightness may develop in certain muscles, affecting how well you can move. This can lead to muscle imbalances and subsequent pain or injury. In one study it was found that many dentists lose flexibility of the neck with side-bending to the left and rotation to the right.[35] These movements are opposite those most used by right-handed dentists.

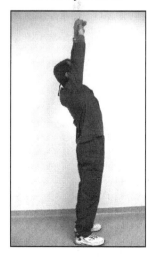

**Fig. 8: Standing with overhead reaching helps to counter back strain due to prolonged, seated postures.**

To prevent low-back pain, it is essential to regularly get out of your chair and assume a relaxed standing posture or stretch.[18] (Fig. 8) Properly designed chairside stretches (Chapter 2) and walking are also helpful in pain prevention. When working positions are confined to a small area, it becomes even more important to perform frequent chairside stretching to counter static postures and prevent muscle imbalances. For optimal low-back pain prevention, avoid remaining in the same position for more than 30 minutes.

Additional strategies to prevent low-back pain include addressing trigger points in the erector spinae and quadratus lumborum muscles, trialing an inversion table (Chapter 8) and improving endurance of trunk stabilizing muscles with specific exercises two to three times a week. (Chapter 9)

> For a free audio (.mp3) download, "Preventing Low-back Pain in Dentistry," please visit *www.posturedontics.com*.

# CHAPTER FOUR

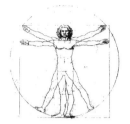

# Dentistry Shouldn't be a Pain in the Neck— or Shoulder

Learning by experience often is painful—
and the more it hurts, the more you learn.

RALPH BANKS

I t's difficult to discuss pain syndromes of the neck without also considering shoulder posture and movements. The neck and shoulder are intimately connected and profoundly influenced by each other via the musculoskeletal and neuromuscular systems. Proper movement in the neck and shoulder is essential to the delivery of dental care and in performing everyday activities.

The incidence of neck pain among dentists and hygienists has been reported as high as 71 percent and 82 percent respectively, with female dental professionals experiencing slightly higher frequencies of pain than their male counterparts.[1,2] Poor posture, movement or imbalances in the neck or shoulder can result in the three most prevalent pain syndromes seen in dentistry: tension neck syndrome, rotator cuff impingement or trapezius myalgia.

Maintaining optimal neck and shoulder musculoskeletal health for dental professionals means understanding the unique muscle imbalances to which you are prone and how various working postures, positions, adjustment of ergonomic equipment and exercise can positively or negatively affect your musculoskeletal health.

# Tension Neck Syndrome

Tension neck syndrome (TNS) feels like it sounds—pain, stiffness and tenderness in the neck and trapezius muscles, often with muscle spasms or tender trigger points.[3] These symptoms may not always be localized in the neck; pain can occur between the shoulder blades or radiate down the arms or up into the base of the skull. Headaches also are a common symptom found with TNS.

Forward head posture is a primary contributing factor to TNS, a problem frequently seen among dentists and hygienists due to years of poor posture involving holding the neck and head in an unbalanced forward position to gain better visibility during treatment. Neck pain has in fact been shown to be associated with any job where forward head posture is 20 degrees or more for 70 percent of the working time.[4] On average, dentists and hygienists work with forward head postures of at least *30 degrees* for *85 percent* of their time in the operatory.[5] Poor endurance of the neck stabilizing muscles can worsen this pain in occupations where forward head postures are required.[4]

Neutral head posture is ear-over-shoulder when viewed from the side. Forward head posture occurs when the natural curve at the back of the neck is put out of balance by the sustained weight of the head (often as heavy as a bowling ball—about 8 to 12 pounds) in the forward position. This can triple the strain on the neck and upper back structures. Recall from Chapter 3 that your pelvic position strongly influences head posture—when the low-back curve flattens, the head tends to move forward. Because of this relationship, the recommendations for maintaining neutral low-back pain posture are largely applicable here.

## Muscle imbalances

Occupations such as dentistry, where forward head and rounded shoulder postures are common, predispose workers to a unique muscle imbalance that is a primary contributor to TNS, thoracic outlet syndrome and numerous other myofascial pain syndromes.[6] This imbalance develops between the neck and shoulder muscles that stabilize and those that move.[7]

The delivery of dental care requires excellent endurance of the primary shoulder girdle stabilizing muscles to maintain optimal posture while performing fine motor skills distally for prolonged periods of time. These muscles tend to fatigue quickly and weaken with prolonged forward head and rounded shoulder posture.[6] (Fig. 1)

**Fig. 1: Shoulder girdle stabilizers (left) tend to weaken quickly with forward head and rounded shoulder postures. Other muscles (right) must compensate and become ischemic and painful**

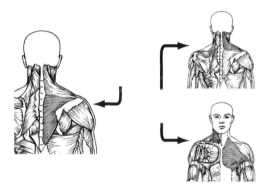

When the stabilizing muscles fatigue, other posterior muscles must compensate, performing postural jobs for which they were not designed. These muscles become overworked, tight and ischemic, resulting in improper movement of the shoulder blade, and neck or shoulder pain.[7]

Meanwhile, anterior "mover" muscles (Fig. 1) become short and tight, further pulling the head forward. Ligaments and muscles eventually adapt to this poor head posture, which can make proper, neutral head postures uncomfortable. The cycle of muscle imbalance perpetuates as tight muscles become tighter and weak muscles become weaker. Because major nerves and blood vessels to the arm run behind these tight muscles, entrapment syndromes may occur as a result of pressure on these neurovascular structures. Since dental professionals are predisposed to this imbalance, discretion is advised when selecting exercises that impact the neck and shoulder. Specific exercises are recommended that target this imbalance (Chapter 9), while certain generic gym exercises may actually worsen this imbalance and pain.

At the end of a career practicing with forward head posture, muscles, ligaments and soft tissue can adapt to this posture and result in permanent postural deformity. You can observe the magnitude of this problem that has befallen many practitioners by observing the startling variety of forward head postures on display from your peers at your next dental convention.

# Cervical Instability

Forward head posture can cause instability in the cervical spine and lead to flattening of the neck curve[8] (especially among women). As muscles, ligaments and tendons stretch, shorten and weaken to adapt to forward head posture, compression on the discs increase, raising the risk of disc injury or herniation. Cervical muscles may spasm and become inflamed as they work overtime to hold the head in unbalanced posture. Once the cervical curve becomes flattened, you will likely need the help of a licensed healthcare practitioner to help restore the natural curve. (Chapter 8)

Cervical instability can also be worsened by performing certain exercises that strengthen the anterior neck and chest muscles.[8] Motor vehicle accidents and whiplash can be debilitating in any job, but especially so in dentistry. The added instability these injuries produce places dental professionals (who are already prone to cervical disorders) at an even higher risk for developing future neck and shoulder problems. Therefore, it is imperative that car accident victims place an especially high priority on all neck and shoulder prevention strategies.

Left untreated, years of forward head posture can lead to cervical spondylosis, a degenerative condition involving osteoarthritis of the cervical spine. In several studies conducted on dentists, the cervical vertebrae have actually slipped forward on each other due to this imbalance. One Finnish radiographic study sampled 119 dentists and revealed that more than half had spondylosis of the cervical spine.[9] The condition has numerous potentially disabling effects, the most notably being compression of the spinal cord, leading to pain, numbness and tingling in the arms and hands.

# Rotator Cuff Impingement

Symptoms of rotator cuff impingement include shoulder pain with overhead reaching, lifting, getting dressed and/or when sleeping on the affected arm.[10] Negligible pain combined with acute weakness may indicate a complete rotator cuff tear.

Rotator cuff impingement causes gradual wearing of the tendon that passes between the humerus and acromion process, due to frequently lifting the arms away from the sides (shoulder abduction) or moving the arm improperly. Muscles that lift or abduct the humerus must be balanced with the muscles that stabilize the humerus in the shoulder joint to allow proper movement (Fig. 2) and help to keep the tendon from becoming "pinched" between the humerus and acromion process.

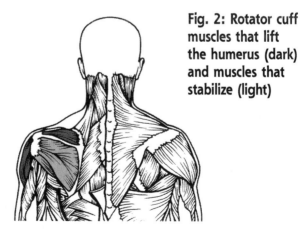

**Fig. 2: Rotator cuff muscles that lift the humerus (dark) and muscles that stabilize (light)**

**Dark Shade:**
Supraspinatus
Deltoid

**Light Shade:**
Infraspinatus
Teres minor
Subscapularis

When properly balanced, the rotator cuff muscles rotate the head of the humerus in the shoulder joint when lifting the arm, keeping it centered and avoiding impingement (Fig. 3A). If the stabilizing muscles are weak, or if the mover muscles become stronger than the stabilizing muscles, it causes the humerus to roll upward into the acromion and pinches the tendon in between, resulting in damage to the tendon. (Fig. 3B)

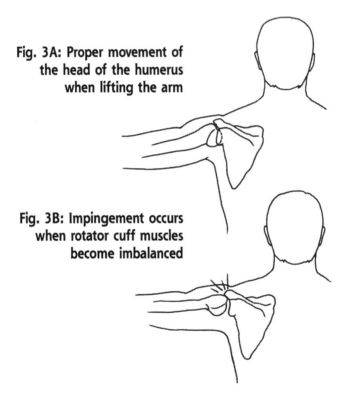

**Fig. 3A: Proper movement of the head of the humerus when lifting the arm**

**Fig. 3B: Impingement occurs when rotator cuff muscles become imbalanced**

Dental-care workers typically injure the rotator cuff via accumulated microtears from overuse due to frequently abducted shoulder postures. The microtears result in instability (muscle weakness) which leads to impingement, which can eventually lead to a complete tear of the rotator cuff tendon. Shoulder abduction beyond 30 degrees can impede blood flow to the supraspinatus tendon, causing ischemia.[11]

(Fig. 4) Dentists and hygienists tend to abduct the left shoulder more than the right,[5] (more than 50 percent of the time) probably due to positioning challenges and using the mirror to retract soft tissue.

**Fig. 4: Lifting the shoulders out to the sides (shoulder abduction) is common in dentistry and can lead to rotator cuff impingement**

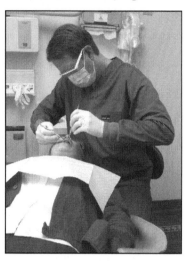

I have observed that shoulder abduction is especially exaggerated in the 10 o'clock position while treating the buccal surface of the upper left quadrant, in the 8 o'clock position when treating large-chested patients, patients who cannot tolerate reclined positions, or when working without a rubber dam.

Excellent endurance and balance of the rotator cuff muscles is imperative to prevent microtears in this tendon. See Chapter 9 for examples of specific strengthening techniques for the rotator cuff. Improper strengthening of the shoulder and chest muscles can easily predispose dental professionals to this syndrome or worsen existing conditions. Ignoring this type of shoulder pain can lead to stiffness, tendonitis, partial rotator cuff tear, and, eventually, a complete tear. Once torn, surgery is almost always required.

# Trapezius Myalgia

The large, flat triangular-shaped muscle between your shoulder and neck is called the upper trapezius. The delivery of dental care places high demands on this muscle and can result in a painful condition called trapezius myalgia. Symptoms include pain, spasms, tenderness or trigger points in the upper trapezius muscle, often on the side of the mirror, or retracting arm. (Fig. 5) Trigger points in these muscles can cause referred pain that extends up one side of the neck as well as referred headaches behind the eye.[12]

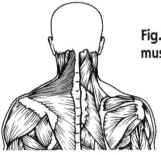

**Fig. 5: The left upper trapezius muscle (shaded)**

The upper trapezius muscles are responsible for elevating the shoulders and rotating the neck. In rounded shoulder posture, the upper trapezius and neck muscles are largely supporting the arm's weight, increasing muscular strain on the neck and shoulder. In dentistry, trapezius myalgia is associated with static, prolonged elevation of the shoulders and, to a lesser degree, abduction of the arms. (Fig. 6)

One EMG study of the neck, shoulders and arms showed that the highest activity during dental work occurred in the trapezius muscles.[13] Sustained low-level contraction of these muscles with few breaks greatly increases susceptibility to pain in this muscle.[14,15] With insufficient rest periods, tension can accumulate in these muscles and, by the end of the day, you may be wearing your shoulders as "earrings" without realizing it.

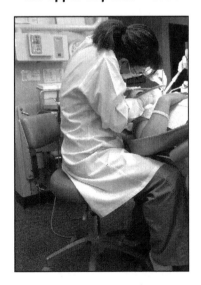

**Fig. 6: Elevating the shoulders can lead to pain, tightness or trigger points in the upper trapezius muscle**

In addition, high levels of emotional stress and working at complex, difficult tasks can cause contraction in this muscle,[14] resulting in ischemic pain.[16] See Chapter 10 for stress management strategies.

Positioning the patient too high or working with the shoulders on a tilted axis or with the head turned to one side or a forward head posture[17] can also lead to worsening of symptoms in these muscles. Since this syndrome is entirely myofascial in nature, it responds well to the muscle therapies in Chapter 8: frequent stretching, heat, massage or trigger-point work.

# Keys to Success:
# Preventing Neck and Shoulder Pain

## *Neutral head posture*

Optimal head posture is ear-over-shoulder when viewed from the side.[10] Since it is nearly impossible for dental professionals to maintain this posture while operating without the use of a procedure or microscope, it is important for them to maintain this postural awareness at all times when not chairside.

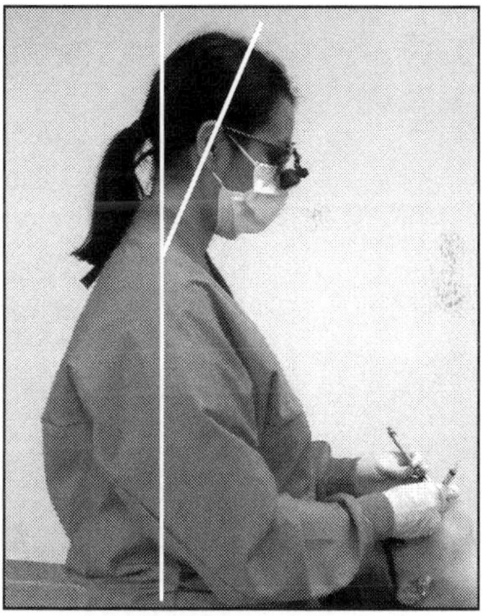

Loupes have been shown to improve operator posture.[18] Since forward head postures of greater than 20 degrees are correlated with neck pain, an optimal head posture of no more than 20 degrees is highly encouraged. (Fig. 7) This will usually require flip-up style loupes. However, due to variations in facial features, some individuals will not be able to attain this posture with dental loupes. Microscopes and procedure scopes allow near neutral head posture (zero degrees) and will be described in Chapter 6.

**Fig. 7: Optimal head posture with loupes is 20 degrees forward**

Neutral head posture has been shown to deteriorate (the head moves forward) with age, probably due to gravity and daily work activities that facilitate this progression. Individuals with chronic neck pain tend to have a poor ability to maintain proper head posture.[19] Since the occupation of dentistry can accelerate forward head posture, it is important to perform postural exercises such as the Dental Postural Awareness Exercise and chin nods (Chapter 2) frequently in the operatory. Chin nods improve endurance of the deep cervical flexors and help maintain neutral cervical postures during prolonged sitting.[19] *Individuals who have sustained injuries in a car accident or have suffered neck injuries should see a healthcare professional before performing any head or neck exercise.*

## *Use armrests whenever possible*

Supporting the arm weight is especially important for trapezius myalgia sufferers.[12] Ensure the armrest height is adjusted properly (Chapter 6). Adjusting the armrests too high can cause neck stiffness and pain at the crook of the neck and shoulder.[12] If you find it difficult to maneuver a chair with armrests around the patient, you may want to consider a unilateral armrest fixed to a counter. (Fig. 8, right) Dentists who operate with the left arm supported have been shown to have less pain than those who do not.[20] These devices are available in a variety of heights and are especially useful since dentists and hygienists experience more pain in the left shoulder than the right.

**Fig. 8: A stool with armrests or a unilateral armrest can be helpful in reducing shoulder and neck strain**

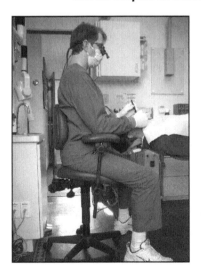
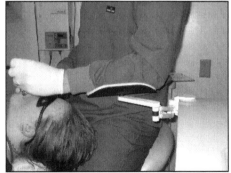

## Neutral shoulder posture and patient height

Neutral posture for the shoulder is often described as elbows at the sides, shoulders relaxed and forearms about parallel to the floor. Helpful advice, indeed—if you are reading a book. This is, of course, an extremely difficult position to maintain constantly during the delivery of dental care. It is far more helpful to know what is a *safe shoulder working range*. The upper arms should abduct out to the sides no more than 20 degrees and reach forward a maximum of 25 degrees.[21] However, when reaching forward further than 15 degrees is required, (due to pregnancy, large breasts or protruding abdomen) armrests are recommended. The occlusal surface should be at, or four centimeters above, elbow level.[21] When the patient is higher than this, arm abduction or shoulder elevation typically occurs, especially when working between the 8 o'clock to 11 o'clock positions.

Operators with short torsos or long upper arms may find that when they position their knees under the patient head or backrest, the combined thickness of the patient chair and patient's head causes them to elevate their shoulders or abduct their arms. This problem is best resolved with a saddle stool, which allows lower patient positioning and improves proximity by opening the operator's hip angle.

## Develop good endurance of specific neck and shoulder girdle muscles

Good endurance of the neck stabilizing muscles is directly related to better neck posture and less neck pain.[4,19,22] Endurance strengthening of the shoulders may also improve neck and shoulder pain, especially among female dentists.[20] All dental professionals can benefit from developing endurance in these muscles, but due to gender differences, it is especially important for women (see "Women in Dentistry" sidebar, page 72). Perform strengthening exercises *only* if you are pain-free and can raise your arm directly overhead and out to the side over your head with little or no pain. (Chapter 9)

## WOMEN IN DENTISTRY

Whoever coined the phrase "my job is a pain in the neck" could have been a female dentist. Compared to the average female worker, female dental professionals experience two to four times more musculoskeletal pain.[28,29] They also report higher frequencies of neck and shoulder pain than their male counterparts. The reasons for this are largely genetic. In general, women's muscles are narrower and can exert only two-thirds the force of a man's,[30] which gives them less ability to counteract unbalanced postures. This is why it is imperative for female dental professionals to target specific muscles in a strengthening program.[31] Bras are also a problem, especially for female dental professionals with large chests. Narrow bra straps can compress the upper trapezius muscle and worsen neck pain and cause headaches.[32] Racer-back sports bras have wider straps and are better suited for female dental professionals. A purse slung over one shoulder can also perpetuate muscle imbalances to which female dental professionals are prone, since the trapezius muscle must contract unilaterally to support the weight.[12] Consider a backpack-style purse, because it distributes weight more evenly.

Women also face modesty issues and some prefer a comfortable distance between their chest and the patient's head. However, positioning oneself farther from the oral cavity shortens the endurance time of the shoulder muscles.[21] This will cause them to crane the neck forward or reach excessively forward with the arms; both are contributing factors for neck and shoulder pain. Armrests can help remove unsafe workloads from the neck and shoulder muscles due to the weight of the extended arm.[22,33-34]

## *Use indirect vision*

Use of the mirror can have a tremendously beneficial impact on neck, as well as trunk posture. Dentists who regularly utilize a mirror tend to have fewer headaches and neck/shoulder discomfort.[2] Side-bending and rotating the neck more than 15 degrees during a majority of one's working hours has been shown to cause damage to the cervical spine.[20] Consider the difference in posture when viewing the lingual upper right area directly vs. using a mirror. (Fig. 9) Lighted mirrors and double-sided mirrors can further improve visibility and ergonomic positioning. (Chapter 6)

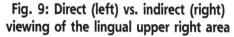

**Fig. 9: Direct (left) vs. indirect (right)
viewing of the lingual upper right area**

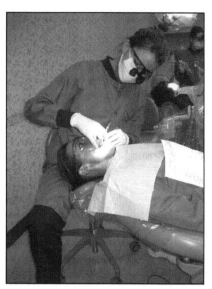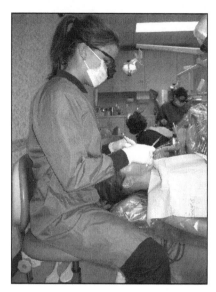

## *Preserve the curve*

It is essential that you preserve your natural cervical curve at night. Consider use of a neck pillow to maintain your cervical curve while sleeping (Chapter 8). Use of a sleeping neck support pillow combined with physical therapy neck exercises has been shown to be an effective combination for chronic neck pain.[23]

## *Periodic stretching*

Both neck and shoulder pain among dentists have been shown to correlate with frequency and duration of breaks.[15] Therefore, frequent breaks and chairside stretching are an important habit to prevent and manage neck and shoulder pain. (Chapter 2) The shoulder circles stretch is especially helpful for preventing trapezius myalgia, while chin nods can improve posture and neck muscular endurance.

# HEADACHES IN THE OPERATORY

### TRIGGER POINTS

A common cause of headaches is musculoskeletal tension in specific neck and shoulder muscles.[12] Headaches that occur frequently (several times/week) and last one to two days are more likely to be myofascial. Trigger point-induced headaches commonly refer pain to the side of the head or face, above or behind the eye or occipital pain.[24] History of whiplash or injuries sustained in a car accident increases the chances that a headache is myofascial in origin.

Poor ergonomics can also predispose you to headaches. Forward head posture has been shown to cause trigger points in the suboccipital muscles, which lead to tension-type headaches.[25] These trigger points may often be self-treated. (Chapter 8)

### STRESS

Depression and stress can cause bruxism and clenching, leading to headaches caused by trigger points in the upper trapezius and the muscles of mastication, especially the masseter and temporalis.[24]

### DIET

Tyramine and sulfites are foods highly associated with migraines and are found in foods like caffeine, red wine, cheese and chocolate. Also processed meats, citrus fruits, lentils, snow peas and monosodium glutamate can trigger headache pain.[26] On the other hand, high-carb foods such as breads, potatoes, pasta, rice and tortillas create a chemical reaction that produces serotonin, a chemical that promotes calmness and helps you deal with stress.[26]

### SLEEP

Control the brain's clock by getting up and going to bed at the same time each day. Too little or too much sleep can contribute to headaches.[27]

### EYESTRAIN

Prolonged focus on an object can cause strain of the eye musculature and blurred vision. Perform the eye-occipital exercise: Frequently focus on an object at a distance. This can be considered a microbreak for your eye muscles and may help counter eye strain related to use of loupes.

# CHAPTER FIVE

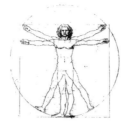

# Getting the Upper Hand on Pain

The right half of the brain controls the left half of the body.
This means that only left-handed people are in their right mind.

SOURCE UNKNOWN

Your hands are integral to your work. Because of sustained grips and prolonged awkward postures dentists and hygienists must employ throughout the day, hand, wrist and arm pain are much more prevalent among these professionals than in the general public.[1] Between 23 percent and 40 percent of dentists experience hand and wrist pain;[2-5] however, among hygienists, the problem is even more prevalent. Nearly 75 percent of hygienists experience hand and wrist pain,[6] which are the most common sites of pain reported among hygienists.[6-9] This frequency is nearly four times the prevalence found in the general working public.

Fewer dental professionals fully recover from hand pain syndromes than they do from pain in the neck, shoulder, and elbow.[7] Therefore, prevention strategies and early attention to warning signs of the primary CTDs of the hand and arm are imperative to your health and career longevity.

One would think that pain in the hand, wrist or arm would be due to a problem in the same area, but the origins of pain are often elusive. In fact, the source of the symptoms may be nowhere near where the symptoms are perceived. For example, one of the symptoms of carpal tunnel syndrome, numbness in the fingers, sometimes has nothing to do with a problem in the hand or wrist, but may be due to a problem in the cervical spine, thoracic outlet or trigger points in the forearm.

There are numerous causes of hand, wrist and arm pain, including tendonitis (e.g., DeQuervain's Tenosynovitis), arthritis (e.g., osteo-arthritis of the basilar joint), nerve compression (e.g., thoracic outlet syndrome, cervical radiculopathy, carpal tunnel syndrome, cubital tun-nel syndrome), trigger points (e.g., Radial Tunnel Syndrome), and equipment issues (non-ergonomic tools, poorly fitted gloves) which will be described later in this chapter. However, the most commonly diagnosed CTD of the hand, wrist and arm among dentists and hygien-ists is carpal tunnel syndrome.

# Carpal Tunnel Syndrome

Carpal tunnel syndrome (CTS) is the most common peripheral nerve entrapment in the arm[10,11] and contributes to one of the most frequently performed surgeries on the hand in the United States.[12] Caused by compression of the median nerve at the wrist,[13] CTS can lead to pain, numbness, or tingling in the thumb, index, middle, and half of the ring finger. (Fig. 1)

One study found that while 71 percent of dentists experienced one or more CTS symptoms, only 7 percent were actually diagnosed with CTS.[14] This should prompt dental professionals with CTS-type symp-toms to educate themselves on all possible etiologies to avoid unnec-essary surgery or ineffective therapies.

Inconsistencies abound in CTS literature regarding its cause, prop-er evaluation and course of care.[15-17] Noted author and physical reha-bilitation expert Dr. Rene Calliet states, "...differentiation of median nerve wrist compression from cervical radiculitis or thoracic outlet

**Fig. 1: Pain or tingling in the distribution of the median nerve (shaded) is often indicative of carpal tunnel syndrome. Numbness is usually felt in the fingertips only.**

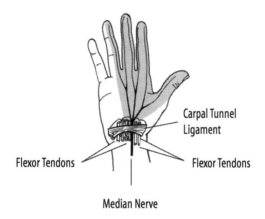

Flexor Tendons · Carpal Tunnel Ligament · Flexor Tendons · Median Nerve

syndrome may be the most challenging in clinical practice."[15] This is largely due to the fact that the median nerve fibers run a long and twisting course around bone and through soft tissue from the cervical spine down to the fingertips. CTS symptoms may not always be indicative of a structural problem in the hand and wrist; often the problem originates more proximally in the muscles/tendons that stabilize the arm during repetitive work.[17] Any compression or entrapment along the median nerve fibers can result in CTS-type symptoms in the hand.[18]

# The Carpal Tunnel

The carpal tunnel is comprised of a row of bones on the back of the wrist, and a thick ligament in the front. For the hand to function properly nine flexor tendons and the median nerve must be able to glide easily within this space, Of these structures, the median nerve is the softest and most vulnerable to pressure.

You can see for yourself the positions that cause the most pressure in the carpal tunnel. Straighten your right wrist and place your left thumb over the transverse carpal ligament. Now bend your right wrist back and feel the ligament tighten over the tunnel. This is the position that compresses the tunnel most. Now make a fist. Did you feel the tunnel get even tighter? If you hold this position long enough, you may eventually feel your hands and fingers go numb. Sustained gripping while extending the wrist is unhealthy for your median nerve. Bring your wrist to neutral, then forward. You will feel the tightness slacken when you are in neutral, then slightly tighten again as you move downward. Now try the above exercise gripping a pencil. This "precision" grip creates more pressure in the carpal tunnel.

You have just demonstrated two of the four primary risk factors for CTS in dental professionals—flexing the wrist forward while gripping a small instrument forcefully. The other two risk factors are high repetition (as in manual scaling) and duration (i.e., how many heavy calculus patients you schedule back-to-back. (Fig. 2)

These risk factors cause microtrauma in the carpal tunnel: fibrosis and edema of the lining of the tendons at the wrist eventually cause increased pressure within the carpal tunnel and decreases the blood flow to the median nerve within the tunnel. The swelling of the lining of the tendons is often painful, and it is the pressure on the median nerve at the wrist from this swelling that causes numbness in the fingers and weakness of the muscles at the base of the thumb.

CTS symptoms (pain, numbness and tingling) are often worse at night and first thing in the morning. Weakness in a precision grip may be present due to atrophy or weakness

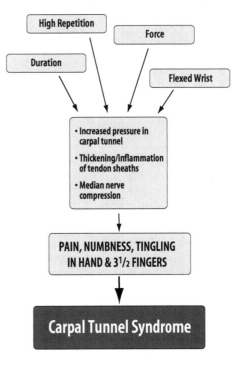

**Fig. 2: Four of the primary risk factors contributing to CTS in dentistry**

High Repetition

Force

Duration

Flexed Wrist

- Increased pressure in carpal tunnel
- Thickening/Inflammation of tendon sheaths
- Median nerve compression

PAIN, NUMBNESS, TINGLING IN HAND & 3½ FINGERS

Carpal Tunnel Syndrome

of the thumb abductor muscles.[19] Over time, visibly decreased mus-culature may be noticed at the base of the thumb. Sensory impair-ment is usually experienced before motor loss, so early intervention is important.

The causes of CTS are numerous and include anatomic, physiolog-ic, hereditary and traumatic factors that result in compression or irrita-tion of the median nerve at the wrist. For instance, CTS is three times more prevalent in women than in men, more common between the ages of 30 and 60, among diabetics and in obese people. However, the literature also reports an occupational cause in more than 47 percent of cases.[20]

In addition to any therapies you may consider, it is imperative that you address ergonomic issues known to aggravate carpal tunnel symptoms. You can use the following strategies in the operatory to minimize your risk for CTS.

# Keys to Success: Preventing Carpal Tunnel Syndrome

The four primary risk factors that contribute to occupational CTS in dentistry can be minimized with appropriate ergonomic interventions.

## *Avoid sustained wrist flexion*

Wrist flexion increases pressure in the carpal tunnel. (Fig. 3, left) Working with your wrist bent toward the little finger—called ulnar deviation—also increases this pressure.[12,13] When you perform scaling or other treatment, try to keep your wrist straight and move your entire hand, wrist and forearm as a unit. This transfers the load from smaller hand muscles to larger arm and shoulder muscles. Using a fin-ger rest position (either inter- or extra-oral) to stabilize the instrument further reduces thumb pinch force and muscle workloads in the hand.[21] Extra-oral fulcrums also facilitate neutral wrist posture and allow proper positioning for precision instrumentation.[22] (Fig. 3, right)

**Fig. 3: Poor (deviated) posture of the wrist is a primary risk factor for CTS in dentistry. Try to maintain neutral posture of the wrist (right), especially when scaling**

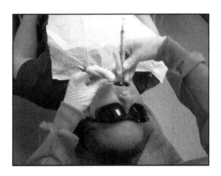 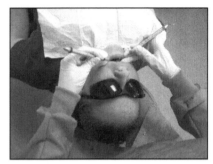

Rather than twisting the wrist to access hard-to-reach areas, try moving the instrument or handpiece in your hand. To access molar regions and distal pockets, select an instrument with multiple accentuated angles and longer terminal shank (Fig. 4), which can reduce twisting the wrist to access these areas. It makes far more sense to use an accentuated angled instrument rather than angling your wrist.

You can retrain yourself to maintain near-neutral wrist postures using a soft wrist wrap, such as a WrisTimer, to limit wrist flexion anywhere from 0 degrees to 20 degrees.

**Fig. 4: Instruments with multiple exaggerated angles and longer terminal shanks can reduce the need to flex the wrist to access hard-to-reach distal pockets**

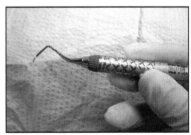

## Go ultrasonic

Compared to manual scaling, use of an ultrasonic handpiece requires less force applied to the work surface and a less forceful precision grip. However, these ergonomic advantages are putting the ultrasonic on the forefront and in some cases overshadowing manual instruments as artifacts of the past. The importance of precision manual scaling in delivering quality dental care cannot be overstated; the effectiveness of quality advanced peri-odontal instrumentation is often hard to match with an ultrasonic unit. Proper ergonomic periodontal instrumentation techniques should be a priority for hygienists to safely implement sufficient hand scaling into their patient care.[22,23]

The percentage of time spent providing ultrasonic vs. manual scaling care is an individual one that must take into consideration personal health (some individuals are more prone to CTS than others), patient perio history, workload, depth and size of pockets and numerous other variables. Both manual and powered instrumentation have unique strengths that can be effectively combined during treatment.[24] Studies show that the *duration* of use of either ultrasonic or manual instruments is positively associated with upper extremity numbness/tingling.[25]

From a preventive perspective, ultrasonic instrumentation should be used periodically over the course of the day to reduce muscle workload and provide rest to the intrinsic hand muscles. Also consider swiveling ultrasonic inserts, which can improve hand and arm posture, as well as save time.

## Instrument selection

Certain instrument features can reduce carpal tunnel compression.

## Diameter

Instruments are available in a wide variety of diameters, ranging from about 5.6mm to 11.5mm. Larger instrument handle diameters reduce hand muscle load and pinch force. However, handle diameters greater than 10mm (about 3/8 inch) have been shown to have no additional advantage.[26] Alternating between handle diameter sizes may help prevent CTS symptoms. When selecting instruments, try to include large diameters as well as other sizes, but avoid the very narrow diameter sizes (5.6mm) which increase carpal tunnel pressure. Sleeves that fit over mirror handles and increase their diameter have been shown to reduce muscle load;[27] however, sleeves on scaling instruments may not have the same benefits due to the additional force needed to perform scaling tasks.

## Weight

Although instrument weight is not as significant a risk factor as handle diameter, lightweight instruments (15 grams or less) help reduce the muscle workload and pinch force.[26]

## Texture

Textured handle surfaces may also help decrease forceful pinch grips.

## Sharpness

Dull instruments can have a profoundly deleterious impact on your musculoskeletal health, as they require increased force. It is essential that you maintain optimally sharpened instruments and perform visual inspections regularly. There are several methods for sharpening, including mechanical, manual[23] or using a high-speed handpiece.[28] (Chapter 6)

## Reduce your grip

Forceful pinch grip has been shown to increase pressure in the carpal tunnel; this pressure is even higher when combined with wrist ulnar deviation.[12] Hygienists and dentists should try to use a palmar grip when using the HVE, and dentists should, of course, use the palmar grip instead of the precision grip during extractions. Dentists with pain in their dominant hand should consider using the nondominant hand intermittently for extractions. Begin by supporting the extracting hand with your dominant hand. As you become more comfortable and transition to using the nondominant hand alone for extractions, you may find that positioning on the opposite side of the patient for extractions is easier and provides yet another opportunity to move around, varying the load on your muscles, bones and joints.

## *Cord management*

Use 360-degree swivel instruments to maintain optimal neutral wrist and finger position. To reduce muscle strain, position heavy cords over your arm through a counter-mounted loop or across an armrest. Prevent cord pullback by positioning your delivery system and ultrasound unit close to you.

Observe patient positioning strategies to maintain neutral wrist posture, as described in Chapter 2.

## *Spread the work around*

Move the muscle workload to avoid structural damage.[29] One way to do this is by alternating between chairs with and without armrests. Using a chair with armrests moves the workload to the smaller muscles of the hand and wrist, while using no armrests incorporates the larger muscles of the arm and shoulder girdle into the movement, as noted in Chapter 6.

## *Temperature*

Another aggravating risk factor associated with CTS is exposure to cold. Avoid positioning your neck, shoulders and hands directly in the draft of an air conditioner or working in a particularly cold environment.

## *Stretch*

Frequent stretch breaks were the most helpful intervention for hand/wrist pain in one dental study.[30] Stretching helps to increase blood flow and reduce formation of trigger points (Chapter 2). If you have mild carpal tunnel symptoms, you should be gently stretching three to five times per day.

# CTS Diagnosis and Treatment

Accurate diagnosis of CTS is difficult and requires evaluation by a highly skilled healthcare practitioner, preferably a board certified hand surgeon. A certified hand therapist (CHT) can also be extremely helpful in addressing adaptation, ergonomics, splinting and using various modalities to reduce your symptoms. Positive results from several tests (EMG and nerve conduction velocity testing, hand pain mapping, sensitivity testing) and presence of wrist/hand pain are highly suggestive of CTS.[12] The following physical exam findings are often seen in people with this syndrome:

- Tinel's sign, an "electric shock" sensation in the hand when the median nerve is tapped gently at the wrist

- Positive Phalen's test. Numbness in the hand in less than 60 seconds when the wrist is flexed 90 degrees

- Weakness of thenar muscles at the base of the thumb

- In severe cases, there may be persistent numbness in the distribution of the distal median nerve (thumb, index finger, middle finger). Continuous numbness can represent permanent damage to the nerve. Surgery should be considered prior to this point, as surgery will reliably prevent further damage to the nerve, but recovery of a damaged nerve is not as predictable.

Conservative treatment options for CTS include:

- Modification of activities to decrease tendon excursion

- Therapeutic interventions such as ice, massage, ultrasound, or acupuncture

- Anti-inflammatories or cortisone injection

- An immobilizing splint across the wrist—often most helpful at night

- Nerve or tendon gliding exercises

- B6 vitamins if the problem is due to a vitamin deficiency

It is advisable to avoid strengthening the hands/fingers with repetitive finger flexion exercises, as this can increase carpal tunnel pressures and worsen pain.[16,31] However, when the patient is completely pain-free, a program of very lightweight tubing exercises focused on the wrist flexor, extensor, pronator and supinator groups may be of benefit in preventing CTS or trigger points.[16]

Dentists and hygienists should implement ergonomic interventions, consider all CTS-mimicking and undergo conservative CTS therapies before considering CTS surgery. Surgical patients treated three to five years after onset of symptoms are less likely to have complete symptom resolution. Therefore, early diagnosis and treatment is important.[12] It is far easier to prevent carpal tunnel syndrome than to cure it.

# Pain Syndromes that Mimic Carpal Tunnel Syndrome

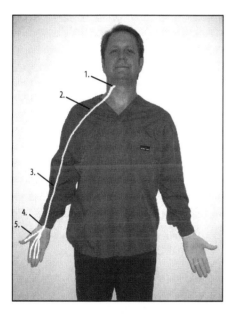

**Fig. 5: Several problems that may mimic CTS:**
1. **Cervical radiculopathy**
2. **Thoracic outlet syndrome**
3. **Median nerve entrapment in the forearm and trigger points**
4. **CTS**
5. **Poorly fitting gloves**

## *Trigger points and nerve entrapment*

Although muscle-referred pain is a well-documented and researched phenomenon,[15,32] it is often overlooked as a possible source of pain syndromes (Chapters 1 and 8). Trigger points in certain muscles may refer CTS-like symptoms into the hand and wrist.[32]

Trigger points in the forearm muscles, such as the pronator teres can cause compression on the median nerve and cause CTS-like pain in the hand and wrist. Since the median nerve runs through the pronator teres muscle, dental professionals, who operate with the hands in a pronated (palms-down) position, are at greater risk for this nerve entrapment.[16,33,34] Neuromuscular technique and myofascial release are two popular approaches that have been used to treat this type of pain. Initially, dental professionals should work with a health-care professional, such as a certified neuromuscular therapist (CNMT) or a therapist who specializes in trigger-point therapy to resolve pain of this origin. After reduction of symptoms, dentists may learn to self-treat their trigger points, since their jobs are a perpetuating factor.[35] (Chapter 8) Median nerve entrapment in the forearm can be treated successfully if a holistic approach is taken to address the sum of compression and tension on the nerves in the upper extremity.[18]

## *Thoracic outlet syndrome*

(TOS) is a neurovascular disorder resulting from pressure on the nerves and/or blood vessels that supply the arm, fingers and hand. (Fig. 6)

**Fig. 6: The thoracic outlet, showing nerves and arteries that supply the arm**

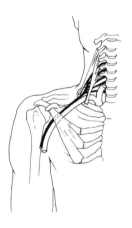

Tightness and/or trigger points in the pectoralis, anterior or middle scalenes may restrict the size of the thoracic outlet.[15,33,36] Compression of this neurovascular bundle may cause numbness and tingling which can mimic CTS. However, TOS may also include vascular symptoms (edema, coldness or discoloration) in the hands and fingers. A thorough clinical evaluation is the most important component for diagnosis of TOS and should include subjective and objective findings, review of daily activities and work habits. The development of TOS has no involvement with the tendons and soft tissues at the wrist, but that is where the symptoms tend to be perceived. In addition to true thoracic outlet syndrome, patients may have thoracic outlet symptoms from forward head posture, working with shoulders on a tilted axis, chest breathing and improper body mechanics.[15,36] Thoracic outlet symptoms from these sources can often resolve with physical therapy.

## Cervical radicular pain

Pain or paresthesia in the hand may also originate in the cervical spine.[15] Nerve roots that supply the arm and hand may become compressed as they exit the spinal vertebrae, resulting in cervical radiculopathy. This may occur simultaneously with CTS (also known as "double crush" syndrome[33]). Numbness in the hand may be produced by changes in neck position, and muscle stretch reflexes tend to be diminished. Electrodiagnostic studies in this situation would reveal a normal nerve conduction velocity; however, the EMG may be abnormal in the distribution of the involved nerve root.[15] A skilled electromyographer, usually a neurologist or physiatrist, is essential for accurate test results. The cause of cervical radiculopathy, more often than not, is due to forward head posture, combined with degenerative changes in the facet joints of the cervical spine.

## Poorly fitted gloves

Improperly fitted gloves may cause CTS-type pain, primarily at the base of the thumb. Ambidextrous gloves are generally molded with the hand in a flat (neutral) position and were originally designed for brief medical examinations.[37] When used for longer procedures, as in dentistry, the operator's hand must pull the glove into a working position, which may compress the back of the hand and strain the muscles at the base of the thumb, simultaneously reducing the blood flow to the hand. Ambidextrous gloves exert one-third more force than fitted gloves.[37] Muscle ischemia, nerve compression and pain may result. Older practitioners may be more prone to glove-related pain in the hands.[38] Tight gloves may also result in the above symptoms.

The cause of hand pain in dental professionals may be multifactorial, and the etiology may not necessarily be related to a single structural problem at the wrist. Regardless of the etiology of hand/wrist pain, dentists should realize that their occupation is a perpetuating factor for the development of this pain.[12,16,32] Prevention is of great importance and intervention strategies should become an integral habit in the operatory, in the office, as well as at home.

# Other Pain Syndromes

## Thumb pain

Osteoarthritis of the CMC joint (base) of the thumb is a common syndrome in occupations with repetitive thumb use and few rest breaks. Therefore, hygienists may be at high risk for developing this disabling syndrome, causing pain at the base of the thumb.

Working with a flattened CMC (proximal thumb) joint can lead to osteoarthritis of this joint, causing stiffness and pain when assuming a forceful pinch grip, as when scaling. Treatment for this condition includes maintaining a flexed CMC joint, avoiding a forceful pinch grip by using large diameter instruments and ultrasonic units, and specific therapeutic exercises.

## De Quervain's syndrome

Hygienists are at greatest risk for this tendonitis, which occurs due to repeated gripping of tools combined with forceful sideways movement of the wrist. A painful tendon inflammation occurs on the thumb side of the wrist that may spread into the thumb or forearm. The pain is usually worse with gripping or twisting movements, and compression from watches and gloves at the wrist can further irritate it. If you suspect you have de Quervain's, try this diagnostic test. Make a fist with your thumb inside so it touches your little finger. Bend your wrist toward the little finger. Mild discomfort is normal. If this reproduces your pain you may have de Quervain's.

Dental professionals should be aware that trigger points in the same muscle that causes de Quervain's tendonitis can refer wrist pain and mimic this syndrome.[39] Prevention and treatment strategies for de Quervain's are similar to those for CTS and include avoiding the irritating wrist motion when possible (see CTS: Keys to Success, page 79), taking frequent breaks, night-time splinting, icing, anti-inflammatory drugs, ultrasound and gentle stretching. A steroid injection into the tendon sheath may give tremendous pain relief, but the injection must be given carefully to avoid injuring a nerve that is adjacent to the inflamed tendons, and some injections can cause skin depigmentation and/or fat atrophy at the site of the injection. Surgery may be indicated if the problem does not resolve. Unlike CTS surgery, de Quervain's surgery has a high success rate if the diagnosis is correct and post-surgery therapy guidelines are followed.

## *Lateral epicondylitis*

Lateral epicondylitis (tennis elbow) is the most common type of elbow problem among dentists and hygienists.[7] It is an inflammation of the tendons that attach at the lateral, bony aspect of the elbow, known as the lateral epicondyle. Pain will be felt when you press directly upon the tendon origin, and when gripping firmly when the elbow is in full extension. The pain is not as much of a problem when gripping with the elbow flexed. The cause is usually the result of repeated upward and inward twisting of the forearm and wrist, especially against resistance. Treatment for true lateral epicondylitis includes wrist stretches, a tennis elbow strap, ice, rest, avoiding the aggravating motion and scheduling wisely to avoid back-to-back heavy calculus patients. Persistent, disabling symptoms can be treated with a steroid injection, and patients who have good but temporary relief of their elbow pain with this type of injection generally do well with surgery.

Trigger points in a forearm muscle can also mimic this pain. Dentists and hygienists are at risk for referred pain from extensor carpi radialis trigger points on the dominant hand.[40] Trigger points in this muscle refer pain to the lateral epicondyle and also to the back of the wrist. These muscles are essential in holding or grasping instruments, when typing, and using "power grips" on hand tools.

Despite all the therapies, drugs and surgeries for hand, wrist and arm pain syndromes, if the ergonomic strain that caused the problem in the first place is not resolved, the condition frequently returns. Make sure you understand and implement appropriate ergonomic interventions in the operatory.

# CHAPTER SIX

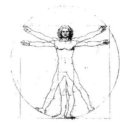

# Dental Ergonomic Equipment

Change is the law of life. And those who look only to the past or present are certain to miss the future.

JOHN F. KENNEDY

Selecting ergonomic equipment that fits your body and your operatory is an important consideration and can profoundly impact your musculoskeletal health. Walk into any major dental conference exhibit hall, and you are quickly inundated with hundreds of product choices and dozens of manufacturers touting their equipment as the best "ergonomic" product of its kind. But how can you tell what products and equipment are the best fit for you and your team?

For new dentists, equipment selection is one of the most critical investments they will make in their careers. Many dentists and hygienists begin to experience pain during their school years,[1,2] partly due to contorting around institutional equipment purchased in bulk, generic quantities for financial considerations. While these units may be adequate for the delivery of dental care, many of them have poor ergonomic design. By graduation, students often have acquired postural imbalances and pain syndromes that they believe simply come with the job and may choose equipment that merely supports a poor posture acquired in dental school.

Dental ergonomic product design has changed over the years, since the advent of seated, four-handed dentistry. For example, many dental stools of the 1960s were a one-size-fits-all design, often just flat, round seat pans with minimal adjustability. Many patient chairs were often designed for patient comfort, rather than operator accessibility. Magnification design has seen drastic improvements from the early clip-on loupes to today's advanced prismatic lenses, microscopes and procedure scopes.

With increasing attention to the high incidence of work-related pain among dental care workers, manufacturers have shifted their focus to ergonomic features. The result is a multitude of "ergonomic" design concepts in the marketplace that can make purchasing equipment confusing for practitioners. Although many dental equipment manufacturers say their products are "ergonomic," they are beneficial only if they adjust to fit your unique body type. What may benefit one operator may not necessarily benefit or accommodate another.

An excellent example of this is ergonomic dental stool designs that feature a very highly contoured seat pan. Due to the pronounced contouring, if the operator's buttocks do not fit the shape precisely, they tend to slide forward, lose proper contact with the backrest, and cannot properly utilize the stool.

Your stature is an especially important consideration in equipment selection. Tall and short doctors require many special considerations with respect to equipment selection: seat pan size, cylinder height, delivery system height adjustment, operatory counter height and magnification working distance, among others.

Dentists and hygienists must understand how ergonomic features impact their musculoskeletal health. Your choices may either improve or worsen your comfort and level of musculoskeletal health. Investing in the wrong equipment leaves you with a dilemma—either replace the equipment (an expensive proposition) or live with it (a painful alternative). Such choices are especially important for new graduates who may be making a large initial investment or for established offices planning renovations.

Ergonomic changes in your office need not involve thousands of dollars in operatory renovation or products. Solutions may be as simple as positioning a patient differently, retrofitting an operator stool with an ergonomic wedge cushion or moving a patient chair within the operatory—all of which cost very little.

This chapter will assist you in understanding how certain ergonomic product features impact your health; how to select, adjust or modify equipment to support your unique body type; and give you the latest research regarding dental ergonomic products. It is also helpful to reference unbiased product reviews in the selection process, though unbiased sources are often difficult to locate. (See "Resources" at the end of this book.)

# Operator Stools

From an ergonomic standpoint, the operator stool is the most important chair in the treatment room. Patients come and go, but you are there all day, so your comfort should be paramount. The seat pan largely influences your pelvic position, which is the foundation of your seated posture. The more neutral your pelvic position, the more balanced your spinal curves become, creating less strain in the back, neck and shoulders. (Chapter 3)

There is a noteworthy difference between chairs and stools. A chair has a backrest and may or may not have armrests. A stool has no backrest or armrests. However, in dentistry, perhaps to avoid confusion between the patient "chair" and the operator "chair," operator seating has been referred to as a "stool." In keeping with this tradition, the word "stool" will be used in this text to avoid confusion.

Historically, operator stools have been designed for average-sized European males. This trend is slowly changing due to the profession's more diverse demographics. (Today, about 70 percent of dental care workers are women.[3]) More manufacturers are offering short cylinder options and short seat pan depths to accommodate this population.

Dentists and hygienists are commonly taught to sit on flat seat pans with thighs parallel to the floor or hips at a 90-degree angle. While this chair design may be tolerable during relaxed sitting, its biomechanical shortcoming is greatly magnified whenever leaning forward is necessary: the combination of thighs parallel to the floor with forward leaning tends to cause the pelvis to roll backward and the low-back curve to flatten.[4,5] Flattening of the lumbar curve has detrimental effects upon both the spinal musculature and discs.[4,6,7] Research suggests that the optimal seated posture for operators is hips higher than knees. (Chapter 3) The increased hip angle decreases muscle activity in the low back, as well as disc pressure. This requires a seat pan design that tilts slightly downward or a saddle-style stool.

Although this may be the most optimal seated posture in dentistry, the recent research on low-back pain and seated biomechanics suggests that there is no single, perfect seated posture.[8] Rather, the spine requires movement to remain healthy. Therefore, a stool that allows frequent spinal movement or readjustment may be beneficial in reducing low-back pain.

Stools that allow dynamic spinal movement while seated may incorporate an air-filled bladder component into the design that follows the operator's pelvic movements.[8] (Fig. 1) Hypothetically, this design may not only reduce low-back pain but also balance the muscle activity in your core stabilizing muscles (between the abdominal and lumbar areas) as well as improve working posture. These designs encourage active sitting but do not constrain the pelvis to one position, as in sitting on a traditional flat seat pan. (Chapter 3) These innovations allow movement of the spine and pelvis by adapting to your body as you move, not vice versa. More research is needed to evaluate the effectiveness of these newer stool designs.

Nontilting seat pans may be retrofitted with a wedge-shaped, air-filled cushion to gain better ergonomic seating and also the benefits of an air-filled seating system. Exercise balls are a common fitness tool used by therapists in building patient's postural core strength. Due to their circumference, these ball chairs may be better-suited for larger operatories, front office, ortho or pedo operatory areas, which typically have larger operating spaces than general dental operatories. Most ball seating systems offer leg extensions to accommodate taller workers.

**Fig. 1: Seating that utilizes air-filled bladders allow movement of the spine, which may help reduce low-back pain**

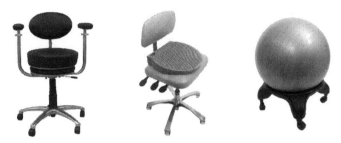

Another way to simulate spinal movement is to alternate between two different seat styles. Consider using a traditional stool (with or without armrests) in one operatory and a saddle-style stool in another. Each design uses very different groups of muscles. Hygienists may switch stools with a colleague mid-morning and mid-afternoon. Also remember to consider intermittently standing for some procedures.

# What to Look For in a Dental Stool

**Fig. 2: Examples of four types of dental stools:
A.) stool with adjustable backrest and seat tilt;
B.) stool with moveable armrests;
C.) stool with adjustable fixed armrests;
and D.) a saddle-style stool**

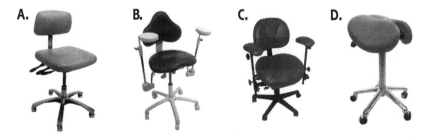

The operator stool should adjust to support your body in neutral back, neck and shoulder posture. (Chapters 3 and 4) With the wide variety of body sizes and heights among dental operators, certain stool types will fit you better than others. Tall and short operators are especially susceptible to pain syndromes due to ill-fitting seating; you should be particularly conscientious when assessing special stool features, as these may benefit or worsen musculoskeletal health.[9] These features include cylinder height, seat depth, stool style and armrests. You should evaluate several styles before purchasing. The following are basic features to evaluate in operator stools.

## Hydraulic controls

Nearly all operator stools today have hydraulic controls for easy, smooth adjustment of the stool. Fewer levers under the seat pan will usually make adjustment easier and quicker.

## Tilting or saddle-style seat

A slight incline of the seat pan (5 degrees to 15 degrees) helps facilitate the lumbar curve in the low back.[10] Tilting seats and saddle-style stools may also enable closer positioning to the patient by opening the hip angle to greater than 90 degrees.

## Seat contour

The seat contour greatly impacts comfort and support. The front edge of the seat should be padded and have a waterfall edge. This feature is especially important when sitting with your thighs sloping downward to reduce pressure on the posterior thigh's blood vessels.

Beware of highly contoured, bowl-shaped seats. These tend to fit only a small percentage of the population. If the operator's buttocks do not fit the contoured shape snugly, they tend to slide forward on the seat and lose contact with the backrest. However, when properly fitted, these styles of seats can provide excellent ergonomic seating in the operatory.

## Seat depth

Dental seat pans range from 14 inches to 18 inches deep and should support most of your thigh. When seated all the way back on the seat and in contact with the backrest, the operator should be able to easily fit at least three finger widths between the edge of the chair seat and the back of the knee. (Fig. 3)

**Fig. 3: Seat pan depth should adequately support the operator's thigh (left); Seat pans that are too deep for the operator (right) may be temporarily modified by angling the backrest forward**

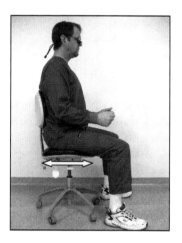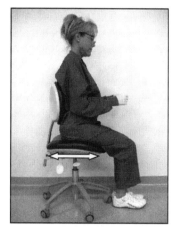

## Seat width

The seat should be wide enough to support the operator entirely. Keep in mind that stools with wider and deeper seat pans require more room around the patient chair for maneuverability.

## Textured seat

The seat's material should be textured to prevent slipping when the seat is inclined forward. Materials such as leather are modern and sleek, but these and certain other synthetic types can be slippery and compromise the stool's ergonomic benefits.

## Backrest

A backrest with good lumbar support helps maintain the spinal curves when sitting.[6] This is an especially important feature with a nontilting seat pan, which tends to flatten the low back curve. Lumbar support helps preserve the lumbar curve, reduces muscle activity disc pressure and reduces back and leg pain.[5,11] Due to the neutral positioning of the pelvis with a saddle stool, a backrest is generally not as necessary.

The lumbar support is the convex portion that supports your low-back curve and need only be eight inches or so in height to provide adequate support. Very large backrests should be carefully evaluated to assure adequate convexity of the lumbar support to properly support the low back and also ensure that the upper portion of a large backrest does not push the thoracic spine forward. The backrest should adjust up and down, as well as forward and backward to support your low back. [*Note*: Use of a prominent lumbar support can worsen pain symptoms among patients with spinal stenosis or spondylolisthesis.]

## Five-caster base on rollers

Five casters are essential for safety. Wide wheelbases are more stable but can be less maneuverable and prevent close positioning to the patient if they hit the patient chair base. Make sure the roller-type is appropriate for your operatory floor (carpet vs. hard floor). The wrong rollers can make it difficult to move the chair around the patient.

## Armrests

Studies support the use of armrests in the prevention of neck, back and shoulder pain.[12-14] Although armrests have been shown to decrease muscle activity in the neck and shoulders of dental professionals, they are not an automatic remedy for all operators with existing neck pain.

Armrests tend to be more popular among dentists than hygienists, since dentists tend to stay in one position longer than hygienists. It may take time to adapt to using armrests, but they can help reduce neck and shoulder pain.

Armrests should be highly adjustable to provide support to the operator in a neutral working posture. Designs vary widely, from fixed, adjustable armrests, to swiveling and telescoping armrests, which move with the operator. Proper height adjustment of the armrest is essential—adjusting the armrest too high or too low can lead to worsening of neck and shoulder pain. Likewise, positioning the armrests too far forward can encourage the operator to lean forward, compromising operator posture. Proper width adjustment between armrests is also important, since armrests set too far apart will cause the user to chronically abduct the arms. You should trial a chair with armrests before purchasing to see if armrests are comfortable and beneficial for you.

## *Cylinder height*

The height of the stool cylinder can significantly impact your seated posture and musculoskeletal health. Stools are sometimes sold with a standard height cylinder with little regard to the height of individual operators. There is no height standardization for dental stool cylinders. Dental stools marketed as average, medium, standard or regular height may vary widely in adjustability, from a low of 13 inches to a high of 30 inches. A "medium" height cylinder from one manufacturer may be called "short" by another manufacturer. In general, it is recommended that a "short" operator have a stool with height adjustment from 16 inches to 21 inches and taller operators from 21 inches to 26 inches.[15] Retrofitting a stool with a short or tall cylinder may allow you to better maximize the ergonomic benefits of the stool.[9]

## *Saddle-style stools*

Operators often ask why a saddle stool is considered ergonomic since it has no backrest. When you are sitting in a horse saddle, your pelvis (the foundation of your seated posture), is in a near-neutral position, as in standing. This pelvic position allows your spinal curves to balance more easily in proper alignment and reduces muscle strain.

This is why backrests are considered optional on saddle stools. By design, saddle stools will place more compression on the peritoneal area, and should be carefully evaluated for suitability to the operator. Due to anatomical differences, some operators will find saddle stools more comfortable than others. Saddle stools are beneficial for several reasons:

- Great for confined areas due to very low profile
- Allow close proximity to patient chairs with thick upper backrests by opening the hip angle
- Easier to maintain your natural spinal curves when leaning forward
- Helpful for tall dentists with low-back pain, since the stools decrease low-back strain

# Patient Chairs

When mulling over a patient chair at an exhibit hall, often the first thing a dentist will do is lie down in it. From an ergonomic standpoint, this is an odd way to evaluate a patient chair. Naturally, you want patients to be comfortable, but the average patient may spend a few hours a year reclined in your dental chair vs. the 2,000-plus hours you spend hovering over it. So whose comfort comes first?

When dental chair manufacturers focus on patient comfort, the result is often a luxuriously cushy chair with wide, roomy armrests. Such designs can create significant problems for you because you must lean or reach over excessive padding to gain access to the oral cavity.

Ergonomics is certainly shifting the focus of these vendors away from the patient more toward you, the operator. But what, exactly, are desirable "ergonomic features?"

# Patient Chair Features

## *Small, thin headrests*

These allow for more legroom and easier, enhanced accessibility to the patient. Large knobs behind headrests can hit your knees or the edge of your stool and should be avoided. Double-articulating and magnetic headrests can allow greater flexibility in patient positioning. Double-articulating headrests can greatly aid in viewing the upper arch when angled up into the patient's occiput. Magnetic headrests allow side-bending of the patient's head to improve access.

## Narrow, thin, upper backrest

Since movement around the patient's head is important to your health, a narrow-profile backrest is desirable. Many patient chairs on the market now have thin upper backrests but are still quite wide through the shoulder area. This inhibits close positioning, especially at the 9 o'clock position. A narrow upper backrest allows for easy movement around the head of the patient, from 9 o'clock to 12 o'clock[16] and will benefit assistants by allowing closer positioning. (Fig. 4)

**Fig. 4: Patient chairs with narrow upper backrests allow easier access**

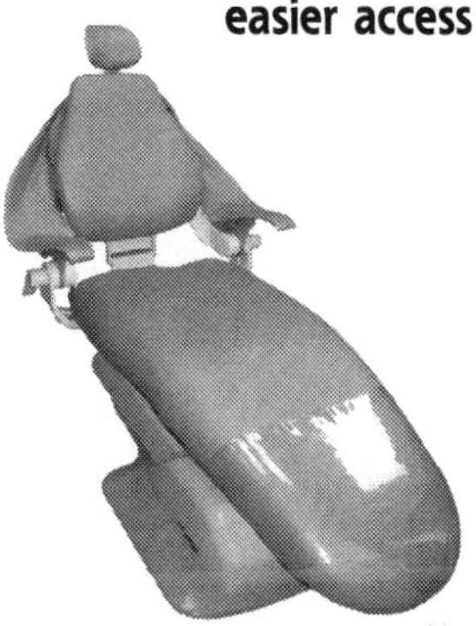

## Sling-style armrests

Sling-style armrests help you to work in the 8 o'clock to 10 o'clock positions without hitting your knees on a fixed metal armrest.

## Height adjustment

The chair should go low enough to allow the dentist to operate in a neutral seated posture. When patient chairs don't adjust low enough, shorter operators are forced to either perch on the edge of their chair or elevate their arms. The chair should adjust high enough so the dentist has the option to comfortably stand for extractions, exams or impression-making without excessive forward bending.

## Swivel feature

The chair should be able to rotate in the operatory to allow access around the patient's head—an important feature if the space between the patient headrest and counter is minimal.

## *Chair length*

Many operatories are small and cannot accommodate certain chair models. Strive for a minimum of 20 inches between the top of the patient chair headrest (when fully reclined) and the counter so you can easily move into the 12 o'clock position.

# Magnification

Telescopes and microscopes have raised dentists' productivity and the level of excellence and confidence in dental treatment.[17] The ergonomic advantages of magnification are increasingly being touted as an important reason to invest in them.

Dental professionals are faced with a unique positioning problem: they must obtain a clear view of the oral cavity while maintaining a static posture for prolonged periods of time. Stress and time demands can cause the operator to lose awareness of body position and compromise their posture. Poor strength of postural muscles can also lead to forward flexed postures, especially toward the end of the day. Properly designed magnification systems can enhance operator working posture by maintaining a set focal range (as with loupes) or by location of fixed binoculars (microscope) or an LCD screen (procedure scopes). Depending on type, magnification supports the operator in head postures ranging from about zero degrees to 25 degrees forward and discourages "postural drifting" forward, thereby decreasing strain on the neck and back.

# Magnification Types

Magnification designs have come a long way in the past decade. Lighter loupe designs with better declination angles have made believers out of many operators who previously purchased loupes, only to abandon them in frustration. As with any ergonomic product, magnification requires proper selection, adjustment, accommodation time and usage to realize their benefits.

There are four basic styles of magnification on the market today: the procedure scope, surgical operating microscopes, loupes (or telescopes) and generic magnification lenses.

# Procedure Scopes

The procedure scope (Fig. 5) offers optimal ergonomic benefits by facilitating neutral spinal alignment and reducing eye fatigue. An extra-oral camera is placed above the patient's mouth, projecting a 1X to 23X image onto a large, flat LCD video screen mounted at eye level directly across from the operator, facilitating neutral posture of the spine. Depth of field is four inches, so the entire mouth can be in focus at the same time. It replaces the exam or procedure light with an LED light with three brightness levels up to 47,000 LUX. It is color-corrected to daylight (5680 Kelvin) to minimize eye fatigue, is cool to touch and radiates no heat onto the patient or staff.

**Fig. 5: The procedure scope is the newest type of magnification and allows the operator to sit upright while viewing images on an LCD screen**

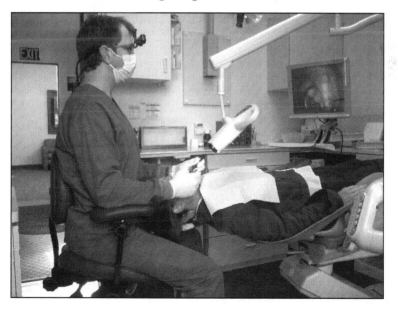

For those who wear eyeglasses, the procedure scope has obvious advantages over units requiring the prescription be ground into a lens. The scope may be ceiling-, counter- or wall-mounted or on a mobile cart. The learning curve is approximately two weeks or more and retails for around $30,000.

# Microscopes

By design, microscopes also facilitate an excellent working head posture, if adjusted correctly, with only zero to five degrees of neck flexion. (Fig. 6) Indirect viewing of the oral cavity is achieved by optics in the scope, which bend the path of the image to almost 90 degrees,[18] allowing an optimal upright posture. Microscopes may be either ceiling-, wall- or chair-mounted and allow a magnification from approximately 3X to 20X.[18] Microscopes are commonly used in endodontics to better visualize and access the root canal system, but they are increasingly being seen in periodontics, prosthodontics, pediatrics and general dentistry to increase efficiency and precision.[19] (Fig. 6) Microscopes use binocular (or infinity) vision, causing minimal eyestrain; loupes, on the other hand utilize a convergence angle which may necessitate an accommodation period, and some fatigue may occur. Additional benefits of microscopes are that the illumination is directed through the optics, so there is no shadowing of the image, and there are no additional weight or cables (as there are in head-mounted loupes illumination).[19] Proper training on the microscope is essential for optimal clinical and ergonomic results.[17] Microscope-users may still find there are situations where traditional loupes are useful from time to time. Asepsis barriers are necessary with both procedure and microscopes, as

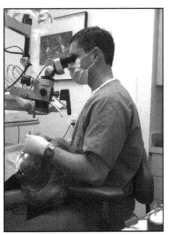

**Fig. 6: Microscopes enable an excellent head posture of only 0 degrees to 5 degrees forward**

the units require manual readjustment. These barriers should be assessed for ease of use in various positions. Lack of portability is also a consideration when purchasing.[20] Prices range from $14,000 to $45,000.

# Loupes

Loupes, or telescopes, are the most popular type of magnification used in dentistry today. While none of these loupe systems provide perfectly neutral head posture (ear-over-shoulder), well-designed telescopes may contribute to clinician comfort[17] and significantly improve operator working postures in dentistry that contribute to musculoskeletal disorders.[21] Because there are some nonergonomic loupes on the market, it is of the utmost importance that the potential buyer be well-educated and prudent in their selection.

Well-designed loupes should enable a working posture of less than 25 degrees of forward head posture. Loupes range in strength from about 2X to 5X and range in price from about $700 to $2,200. Two basic styles are on the market: through-the-lens (fixed mounts) and front lens mount (flip-ups). (Fig. 7A & B)

## *Through-the-lens (TTL) loupes*

- Scope is mounted into the lens
- Wider field of view, since scope is closer to the eye
- Do not get knocked out of adjustment
- Declination angle is preset and not adjustable
- Slightly lighter weight than flip-ups
- Changes in eyeglass prescription lenses require return to manufacturer for modification

**Fig. 7A:**
**Through-the-lens loupes**

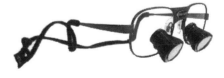

## *Flip-up loupes*

**Fig. 7B:**
**Flip-up loupes**

* Scope is mounted in front of the lens, generally on a hinge mechanism

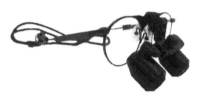

* Better declination angle for optimal head posture

* Can sometimes get knocked out of adjustment

* Tend to be slightly heavier

* Loupe can be easily flipped up when not in use

* Eye-glass prescription can be easily changed by local optician

Prescriptions can be built into the carrier (larger) lens in either type scope for distance viewing. In flip-up styles, the carrier lens can also have a bifocal prescription. With TTL styles, the actual scope may have a prescription. Some loupe manufacturers have a maintenance program that allows bi-yearly prescription changes for a one-time fee.

# Generic Lenses

Generic lenses may come in frames or clipped onto prescription glasses, are the most economical and have been with the profession for decades. These are generally low-magnification (2X); some models may be purchased over the counter. Generic lenses (or "reading glasses") give approximately the same view of the oral cavity as when you hunch over the patient. Unfortunately, there is minimal ergonomic benefit, since there is usually no declination angle feature, causing the operator to tilt the head forward to operate.

# Loupes Lingo

The three most important ergonomic factors to consider when purchasing loupes are declination angle, working distance and frame size.

# Declination angle

The angle that your eyes are inclined downward toward the work area is the declination angle. (Fig. 8) This angle should be steep enough to help you attain a comfortable working position with minimal forward head posture (less than 25 degrees).[22] The farther the head is positioned forward to see through the loupes, the greater the strain on the neck muscles and discs.[23,24] A downward declination angle that is too extreme can theoretically cause eye strain;[24] however, the author has rarely observed this problem clinically. By far, the predominant problem observed regarding declination angles are insufficient (small) angles that force the operator to assume unhealthy working postures.

Since glasses rest differently on each face, the same pair of loupes may have a slightly different declination angle from one person to the next. The declination angle can vary dramatically and can either benefit or worsen musculoskeletal health. Generally, flip-up style loupes allow a steeper declination angle and more neutral head posture compared to TTL loupes. Therefore, it is a good idea, when ordering TTL loupes, to request the *steepest declination angle possible*.

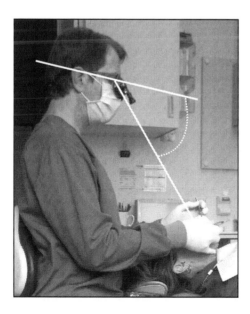

**Fig. 8: Telescopes with a good declination angle (white lines) allow the operator to work with minimal forward head posture**

# Working distance

The working distance is the distance from the eyes to the working area. If the working distance is measured too short, it can result in excessive neck flexion or hunching.[25] At convention booths, mounted typodonts cannot take into consideration the thickness of your own patient chair or your preferred working height. A discrepancy of just a couple of inches can have a significant impact on your comfort and health.

It is better to measure the working distance in your own operatory, with a patient in the chair. Sit in neutral operating position and find your preferred position within the recommended postural working range. (Chapter 2) Have someone view you from the side and measure the distance from your eye to the work surface, or tooth. Working distances will vary for shorter operators (14 inches or less) to extra-long working distances for very tall operators (more than 20 inches). Working distance should be tailored to the individual.

# Scope position

Keep in mind that the lower the manufacturer can place the scope in relation to your pupil, the better working posture you will usually have. Large frames that sit low on the cheek will allow the lowest placement of the scope. (Fig. 9) In general, flip-up scopes will sit lower in relation to the pupil than TTL scopes.

Even when ordering a large frame, some manufacturers may not mount the scope as low as needed. It may be helpful, especially when ordering TTL loupes, to verbally request that the scope be placed as low in the large frame as possible.

The nosepiece adjustment can also have a significant impact on how high the frames sit on the face, and can therefore affect the height of the scope in relation to the pupil. Widening the nosepiece will often allow lower placement of the frames on the face.

**Fig. 9: Large frames generally allow for lower positioning of the scope in relation to the pupil, which usually enables a better working posture.**

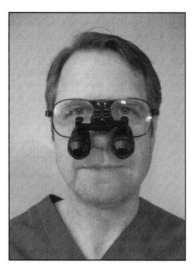

# Selecting Telescopes

Products are often designed for the "average" individual—a person who does not exist. Everyone is a deviation from the norm. Interpupillary distance and nose bridge height will affect how certain scopes fit you. Therefore, it is important to try on several brands and styles to determine which fits you best. Although dental conventions provide a good opportunity to do this, if possible, you should bring the working distance measurement that was obtained in your own operatory with your own equipment.

General guidelines for magnification strength are as follows: for hygienists, 2X to 2.5X; for general dentists, 2.5X to 3.5X; for endodontists/periodontists, 3.5X to 4.5X or higher. In general, operators should start with the lowest magnification at which they can view and control the surgical field, although personal prescriptive factors and optical conditions may affect this recommendation. Keep in mind that higher powered scopes will create a shorter depth of field, which may make working in multiple areas of the mouth difficult. Work with your local scope representative to ensure proper measurement, adjustment and working posture. It is not unusual for new loupes to need slight adjustments, so be sure to evaluate your new scopes carefully, and do not hesitate to contact the manufacturer's technical support for adjustments as necessary.

# Adjustment Period

I've consulted with many operators who have tried loupes but say they could not get used to them. Just as incorporating any new equipment or procedure into the practice involves a learning curve and requires some patience, scopes are no exception. Initially, wear your new loupes for no longer than a couple of hours for the first few days, and gradually increase your wearing time over a 5- to 10-day period to become accustomed to the new acuity, posture and field of vision that magnification offers. Speeding this process can lead to headaches. Your manufacturer representative should work with you to resolve any problems with adjustment and comfort following your purchase.

# Lighting Systems

Overhead lighting can be inadequate because you or your assistant may be in positions that block it from the mouth and cast shadows over parts of the working area. Many dentists find that overhead lighting, even in combination with fiber-optic handpieces, provide inadequate illumination.

When considering options to light the oral cavity, it is helpful to understand illumination terminology. Lux (LX) is the unit of measurement most commonly used; however, foot candle (ft c) is an older term that is still in use today. One foot candle (equal to 10 lux) is approximately equal to the light emitted from one candle 12 inches away. It is important to avoid extreme contrast between the ambient light and task light. For optimal visual acuity and comfort, past recommendations have suggested that the task, or spot lighting area, be three times brighter than the ambient lighting.[26] However, Dr. David Ahearn, president of Design Ergonomics Inc., points out that with today's higher-powered dental lighting systems, this ratio would cause the room to be unbearably bright. Spot illumination in dentistry ranges anywhere from 18,000 lux to 38,000 lux, and recommendations for ambient lighting in a room with high-precision work is 1,000 lux to 2,000 lux.[26] If one were to follow the 3:1 ratio, this would mean ambient operatory lighting of 6,000 lux to 12,000 lux, which far exceeds ergonomic recommendations.[26] You will also need to consider other factors when determining your optimal ambient lighting in the operatory, such as type of overhead lighting, reflectance of work surfaces, and amount of natural lighting.

You have several options to enhance illumination of the oral cavity. Mounted headlamps attach either directly to your scope frame or separately to a head strap. Lamps are powered by plug-in units with fiber optic cables or by smaller portable battery packs that can be carried between operatories. The smaller powered units have traditionally not provided strong enough lighting, but newer LEDs and improved rechargeable batteries deliver better performance. Current models have the added advantage of being lighter in weight.

It is important to note that these additional head-mounted light sources also come with caveats. Some increase in neck strain may occur due to the weight of some models. Fiber-optic cables add more weight and can snag on chair levers and knobs. Considerations when purchasing lighting include intensity (lux), spot size, weight, color temperature and battery life.

Dryfield illuminators allow the practitioner to isolate quadrants of the mouth and direct light where it is needed. They also provide aspiration of debris and fluid, and retraction of the tongue and cheeks. New designs have fiber-optic cables and suction combined (instead of in separate tubes), minimizing the inconvenience of tubes stretching across space or cabinetry.

# Rubber Dams and Lip/Cheek Retractors

These aids may also assist the operator in reducing neck and shoulder strain by reducing the need for the assistant or dentist to manually reflect slippery cheek tissue. I feel this elevates the much maligned and underutilized rubber dam as a primary piece of ergonomic equipment by allowing operators to better use indirect vision. Rubber dams also preclude the need to constantly struggle against soaked cotton rolls and flopping tongues, and they prevent saliva contamination of the working field.

# Manual and Ultrasonic Scalers

Both manual and powered instrumentation have unique strengths that can be effectively combined during treatment. See Chapter 5 for an in-depth description of ergonomic impact and selection guidelines for each.

## *Sharpeners*

Sharpening may be performed by the hygienist or a specially trained assistant, using either manual or mechanical sharpening techniques. Three popular methods for sharpening include mechanical, manual and high-speed handpiece. Most hygienists are taught manual sharpening in school; however, it may be difficult to obtain exactly the correct sharpening angle using this technique. Mechanical sharpeners require less muscular effort but are more expensive. Another method of sharpening instruments is using a high-speed handpiece.[28] It is important for accuracy that magnification is used to visualize the cutting edge. Regardless of the method used, proper training is advised.

Scalers are now available made from materials that hold a sharp edge much longer than older scalers. When considering scalers that need no sharpening, keep in mind the life of the instrument, which may be only three to four months before it must be discarded.

# Gloves

Ambidextrous gloves may cause carpal tunnel syndrome-type pain, especially at the base of the thumb. (Chapter 5) Ambidextrous gloves are generally molded with the hand in a flat position, whereas fitted gloves are molded with the hand in a more dynamic working position.

Gloves that are too tight may also cause pain. A general guideline for fitting gloves is that they should be loose across the back of the hand and palm to aid comfort and circulation and snug in the fingers to improve touch acuity.

The proper selection and adjustment of ergonomic operatory equipment plays a key role in the management and prevention of work-related pain in dentistry. Since dental equipment technology is constantly changing and advancing, dentists and hygienists should visit trade shows to gain knowledge of the most recent offerings in these areas.

# CHAPTER SEVEN

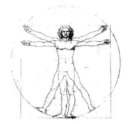

# Operatory Layout and Systems

He that will not apply new remedies must expect new evils;
for time is the greatest innovator.

SIR FRANCIS BACON

T he design and selection of treatment rooms should be geared toward the comfort, health and productivity of you and your staff. These three objectives are, on occasion, in conflict with one another, and thus careful planning and consideration must be given to all of the choices at hand. It will be important to have a clear sense of your priorities before implementing a design and equipping plan. Here are some examples of the necessary tradeoffs and decisions you are required to make as you plan a layout. Do you want to maximize the room capacity of your office or do you want more storage? Do you want a more visible and thus potentially threatening (to the patient) layout, or can you create a layout that will reduce patient anxiety? Should you optimize your layout for four-handed dentistry or do you need to accommodate successful two-hand function?

The decisions you make will have a significant impact on your practice health and success.

Be sure to consult the resources at the end of this book for four-handed dentistry techniques, transfers and dental office design consultants. For the purposes of this book, we will focus on those considerations that impact operator posture and body mechanics, including delivery systems, counter height, patient chair orientation, assistant delivery systems and computer systems, but we will not touch on all aspects of overall room design.

# Delivery Systems

Rear, side, over-the-patient or over-the-head delivery—which of these is right for you? While manufacturers frequently tout the esthetic and productivity features of different delivery systems, there is a paucity of literature regarding both the impact of each type on dentists' musculoskeletal health or on actual productive capacity. Each delivery system has its advantages and disadvantages. Understanding these can help you select the right system for your team.[1]

From a productivity standpoint, the assistant's ability to function with your delivery system should be a primary consideration. This is very often overlooked when doctors select room options at the trade show or dealer showroom. Assistants should be able to easily retrieve suction, syringes, instruments and, possibly, handpieces. This enables you (or the hygienist, if using assisted hygiene) to operate without shifting your field-of-view to retrieve instruments or handpieces or to change burs. The most frequently used handpieces should be placed closest to the assistant. It should be noted, however, that handpiece use actually compromises no more than 15 percent of a typical procedure, thus their placement ergonomically is of far less importance than that of the entire treatment arrangement.

Hoses on all delivery systems should be lightweight and flexible to avoid muscular strain. This is usually achieved with silicone, low voltage, straight six-pin or ISO-C tubing. Although fiber-optic bundles have better light output, they also add weight and rigidity.

# Rear-Delivery Systems

Rear-delivery systems accommodate all clinical instruments behind the patient, which frees up space for other, larger pieces of equipment in the operatory. It is the least expensive way to connect to utilities and keeps the equipment out of view of the patient, which decreases anxiety. Functionally, rear delivery works fairly well when true four-handed dentistry is practiced (i.e., equipment is within reach of the assistant, who transfers instruments, retrieves handpieces and changes burs).[2]

However, rear delivery is the poorest method of delivery in two-hand function. More often than not, rear-delivery systems encourage operators to extensively reach, lean or twist their torsos to retrieve instruments from behind the patient's head (Fig. 1), which can contribute to low-back pain.[3,4] Operators should try to retrieve instruments with the closest (nondominant) hand to avoid repeated twisting or reaching across the body (Fig. 2) and then transfer the instrument to the dominant hand.[5] If rear-delivery rooms are designated for even a moderate amount of two-hand use, they should be reconfigured to an alternative delivery system.

The ability to frequently reposition and move around the patient's head

**Fig. 1: Operators should avoid repeatedly twisting to one side to retrieve handpieces from a rear-delivery system**

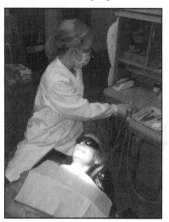

**Fig. 2: Operators with rear delivery should retrieve instruments with the nondominant hand and transfer the piece to the dominant hand**

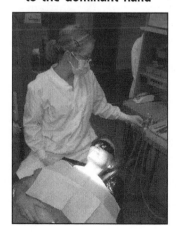

is imperative to your musculoskeletal health.[5] Some rear-delivery systems limit access from 11 o'clock to 12 o'clock positions, which generally offers the best ergonomic access during a procedure. In addition, when positioned from the 7 o'clock to 9 o'clock positions, it is difficult, if not impossible, to reach the rear-delivery system without leaning or extended reaching (a risk factor for neck and shoulder pain). Therefore, rear delivery may limit your movement around the patient.

# Side-Delivery Systems

When placed correctly, side-delivery systems require less trunk-twisting for the doctor than rear delivery to retrieve instruments. (Fig. 3) However, since the assistant cannot reach the instruments, the dentist must remember to squarely face the system when changing burs, rather than sustaining a twisted posture.

**Fig. 3: A well-placed side-delivery unit minimizes leaning and twisting but decreases effectiveness of the assistant**

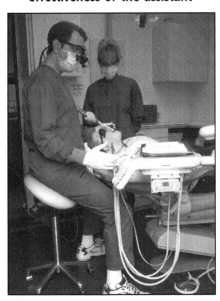

The main ergonomic concern I see with dentists who use side delivery is the tendency to lock themselves into one working position relative to the patient, hour after hour, day after day.[5] This tends to overwork and fatigue certain areas of the body and can lead to pain. The best practice with any delivery system is to change positions as frequently as possible during procedures.

Proximity of the system is also a concern. Often, as operators move around the patient's head, they do not reposition the side-delivery system and repeatedly lean or twist to one side to retrieve instruments. Keep in mind that, from a resale perspective, most side-delivery units are not interchangeable for left-right handed dentistry.[2]

Also, since the dentist is retrieving the handpieces and the assistants cannot reach them, productivity is often compromised. There is an emerging concern with side delivery as it relates to high technology. Side-delivery units obstruct the egress of equipment, such as lasers and CAD/CAM units, in the operatory, a problem likely to increase over time as more and more capabilities emerge.

# Over-the-Patient Systems

Over-the-patient (OTP) delivery systems allow you to move freely from the 8 o'clock to 12 o'clock positions around the patient's head. The unit is located over the chest of the patient, so handpieces and other instruments are within easy reach for both you and your assistant, minimizing your movement and shift of vision. (Fig. 4)

However, this system is highly visible and in close proximity to the patient. It may also be bumped by the patient, which makes it especially undesirable for most pedo offices.

**Fig. 4: Over-the-patient delivery systems allow freedom of movement around the patient's head but may require upward reaching**

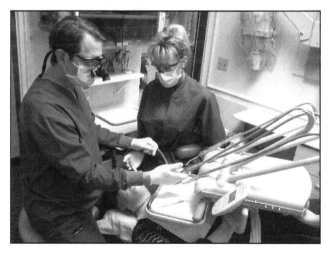

The design may be less ideal for operators with short torsos. When it is placed over a large patient, shorter operators may be forced to repeatedly reach upward for instruments, risking neck and shoulder pain.[5] Using a microscope with OTP delivery may compromise access to the delivery system at the 11 o'clock and 12 o'clock working positions. This problem can be reduced through the selection of a unit with long arms that will permit the unit head to be located beside the patient. Unfortunately, in so doing the problems of side delivery come into play. Also, for your assistant's health, don't position the system too far down the patient's stomach, since this will cause your assistant to have to twist to retrieve instruments. These systems can be designed to convert flexibly with right-left handed adjustability, which not only impacts ergonomics, but also helps in the resale of your practice, specifically for left-handed dentists who are likely to find a right-handed buyer. Should right-left convertibility be a significant objective, make sure that the rest of the operatory is designed to support this goal.

# Over-the-Head Systems

Over-the-head delivery systems have recently become recognized as a unique solution to dental delivery.[1] (Fig. 5, left) Combining many of the benefits of over-the-patient and rear-delivery systems, over-the-head sys-

**Fig. 5: Over-the-head delivery, due to its forward position, permits the doctor and assistant full access to all supplies**

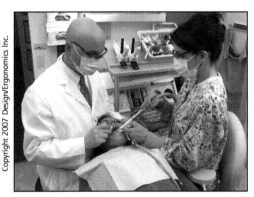
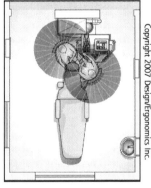

Copyright 2007 Design/Ergonomics Inc.

Copyright 2007 Design/Ergonomics Inc.

tems afford the operator the ability to practice from the 7 o'clock to 1 o'clock positions. (Fig. 5, right) Supplies are in an ideal position for assistant access, while handpieces are more accessible than rear-delivery layouts, reducing the ergonomic challenges when in two-hand function.

Additionally, over-the-head layouts, when properly configured, convert from right- to left-hand function rapidly.

# Operatory Layout

Advancements in dental technology have been a boon to the profession. But there is ever more dental gadgetry to try to fit into small operatories. Imagine trying to fit Wal-Mart's stock into a 7-11 store—all within easy reach. Okay, this is stretching it, but you get the idea. Trying to find room for the ever-increasing array of products in a small operatory is a major ergonomic challenge. The primary objectives are to identify the equipment used most frequently, such as dental instruments, supplies and handpieces, and to place those within easy fingertip reach.[6] Equipment used less frequently can be placed farther away or mobilized for room-to-room sharing. Proper placement of equipment can be determined by sweeping the forearm in a horizontal arc, with your elbow relaxed at your side. All frequently used equipment should be within this radius, which is about 14 inches to 18 inches from the elbow. This process applies to both doctor and dental assistant. Lesser-used equipment should be placed no farther than 25 inches from the shoulder when the elbow is extended.[7] (Fig. 6)

**Fig. 6: An ideal operatory configuration will place all of your commonly used supplies within fingertip access**

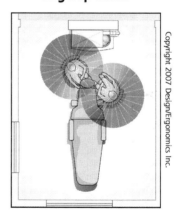

Copyright 2007 Design/Ergonomics Inc.

Dental office design expert, Dr. David Ahearn, president of Design Ergonomics, emphasizes the importance of operatory layout and consolidating primary working areas to increase productivity and decrease unnecessary motion. Increases to productivity are significant when an environment is created that minimizes range of motion and non-value-added steps in the delivery process.[6]

A well-designed operatory also will be equipped for quick conversion from one type of procedure to another. One of the best ways to accomplish this is to set up high technology for rapid mobilization.[8]

The position of the dentist and assistant during treatment can also have a significant impact on productivity as well as musculoskeletal health. Four basic doctor/assistant treatment positions should be evaluated by the dentist and assistant for its appropriateness in their office. (Chapter 11)

# Counter and Delivery System Height

To prevent neck and shoulder dysfunction, the height of the oral cavity, counters and delivery system should be at about elbow height when the operator is seated with arms relaxed at the sides.[7] This is much lower than typical counter height. Fixed-height rear-delivery systems and counter height can be a problem for both tall and short operators. Fixed rear-delivery systems used by short operators are especially problematic, since many fixed systems were designed for the average-sized man. On the other hand, I have seen dentists 6 foot, 5 inches and taller have to bend over to retrieve items from a standard counter height of 32 inches. The best way to reduce height-related compromises is actually to reduce the distance to reach implements. One solution for taller dentists may be wall-mounted cabinets that do not extend all the way to the floor.[2]

Ideally, when you and your patient are positioned at the proper height (Chapter 4), the delivery system height, counter height and oral cavity are approximately at the same level. Tall or short operators often need to modify existing counters or delivery systems.

A short dentist or hygienist sharing operatories with a tall dentist or hygienist can be an ergonomic nightmare. Adjustable height on patient chairs, delivery systems, stools and armrests can help, but only to a certain point. When operator heights vary dramatically, it is often best for operators to purchase their own stools with tall or short cylinders. Patient chairs and delivery systems can then be adjusted accordingly.

# Assistant Delivery Systems

Fixed counters are frequently used as the assistant's work surface and are frequently located too far away from the assistant, causing excessive reaching. Swiveling the patient chair often allows the assistant closer positioning to the fixed counter. Moving the patient chair closer to the rear counter may also be required.

The most ergonomic assistant delivery system is a *movable* work system, because it allows assistants in a variety of sizes and heights to use the unit. Movable systems should have right- or left-handed adjustability, be height adjustable and extend over the assistant's lap. These systems are wall-, cabinet- or cart-mounted and should be adjustable in all planes. Wall systems are easily installed but often lack the necessary adjustment cabinetry to allow them to function without excessive bending or twisting or even forcing the assistant to leave her position to retrieve supplies.

Cabinet-mounted systems are widely available and generally increase the level of adjustability; however, this adjustment is limited to one or two axes. When choosing a cabinet system it is imperative that the counter section have the ability to pull out over the assistant's knees, enabling full accessibility to utilities from the seated position.

A common type of assistant delivery is a mobile cart, which is a unit on wheels that can move freely in the operatory. It may have multiple storage drawers in front or simply an open U-shape frame. (Fig. 7)

**Fig. 7: Assistant mobile carts offer less ergonomic flexibility but may be a more economical solution**

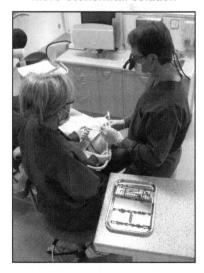

Either type should have a surface that extends over the assistant's lap.[2] These mobile units are often an effective, inexpensive ergonomic modification for certain operatories. However, there must be adequate room to place the cart while still maintaining the assistant's optimal position chairside, which is assistant hip at patient's shoulder. (Chapter 11)

# Utilities

Suction and air-water syringe systems are important aspects of the delivery system. Utilities that are placed behind the assistant cause excessive twisting. (Fig. 8) These may sometimes be remounted with

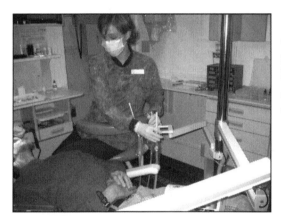

**Fig. 8: Suction and air/water syringe systems located behind the assistant cause excessive twisting**

**Fig. 9: Suction and air/water syringe system remounted on arm extended in front of assistant**

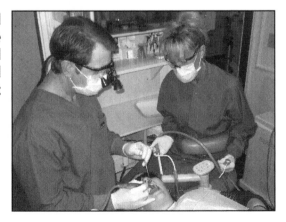

an extended arm, allowing retrieval from in front of the assistant. (Fig. 9) This will largely depend on patient chair type. Unfortunately, this pushes the assistant back from the patient—a compromise that doctors would not accept for themselves. When possible, position the utilities to avoid blocking the assistant from close proximity to the patient.

Lighting should usually be adjusted by the assistant. The light track and joints should glide smoothly and require minimal effort to reposition. The light handle should be oriented vertically, since this is the safest biomechanical position for the shoulder.

# Patient Chair Orientation

Orientation of the patient chair in the operatory can greatly affect operator posture and body mechanics. Of the utmost importance is that there be at least 20 inches of space behind the patient chair to allow the operator to work at the 12 o'clock position.[2] As noted in Chapter 4, the 12 o'clock position enables one of the most neutral operator working postures. If this position is not attainable, try swiveling the patient chair 15 degrees to 20 degrees to access the 12 o'clock position.

Remember that the patient chair is usually not a stationary fixture in the operatory, but can often be moved several inches, depending upon where the electrical box is located. Moving the chair farther from or closer to the counter or angling the chair within the operatory can often improve ergonomics for all team members.

# Computer Technology

From computers to radiography, digital technology has become a common feature in many operatories. Computer, monitor and keyboard placement are important considerations that can impact team members' health. Computers should be placed out of the patient's view in a cabinet, if possible.[9] Side- and rear-delivery cabinetry offer ideal locations for these. If there is not sufficient room to hide a computer box or run computer cables, consider an all-in-one system, where the computer is built into the screen and controlled by a keyboard/mouse in an ergonomic location. Another option is a laptop computer; however, laptops are difficult to keep clean, which may pose an asepsis problem. In general, when compared to PCs, both laptops and all-in-ones tend to be more expensive, are usually less powerful and must be sent in for repairs. If you are considering integrating other technology into the operatory, such as a camera, you may require space for add-in cards. PCs typically have two to three slots available, the all-in-one has one slot, and the laptop has none.[10]

Consider systems that adjust to support the operator's optimal position. These include arms that swing in toward the operator, then move easily out of the way when not in use.

Monitor placement is extremely important from an ergonomic perspective. Ideally, there should be two monitors in the dentist's operatory: one placed behind the patient for the assistant and/or clinical staff and one in front of or above the patient.[11] In general, the position of a monitor at a close range should be at a height where the top of the screen is at or slightly below eye level. Consider a flat-screen monitor whenever possible. The assistant's monitor can be located behind the patient (in the 12 o'clock to 2 o'clock position) and can show patient records and HIPAA-sensitive information since it is outside the patient's view. The patient/dentist monitor can be used to show camera images, x-rays or patient-education videos. Location of this monitor varies, depending on the operator's preference. Higher placement of the patient monitor (as in pole- or ceiling-mounted) will allow the operator to fully recline the patient while still allowing easy viewing of the monitor.[9] If the operator wishes to use the second monitor for diagnostic and patient education purposes, the monitor/screen may be located at the 9 o'clock position on an arm that is long enough to reach in front of the seated patient.[10] (Fig. 10) This allows patient education in a more personal manner, without requiring the dentist to turn their back on the patient while addressing a different screen.

When monitors are positioned closely enough, consider touch panels, as it is more intuitive for someone to point to something, rather than play "follow the cursor."[10] For monitors positioned farther away, a Gyro mouse is a good option, as it can be held in any position and does not need a surface. Screen size will depend on location—at greater dis-

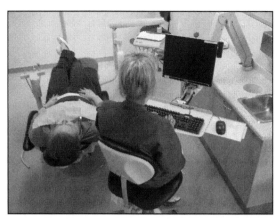

**Fig. 10:
The operator's
computer can
be mounted
in a variety
of locations,
depending upon
desired use**

tances, a larger screen will be needed. A good rule of thumb is that at 2X the distance, you will need a 4X larger screen to have the same detail. In other words, a 15-inch monitor looks the same at 2 feet as a 30-inch monitor does at 4 feet.[10]

The keyboard should be located at a height where the operator's forearms are parallel to the floor or sloping slightly downward. Achieving both ideal keyboard *and* monitor height are difficult with a laptop computer. Look for a keyboard that has a built-in mouse, such as a trackball or touchpad. A wireless keyboard expands positioning possibilities.[9]

Due to the unique nature of each operatory, I recommend contacting a dental technology specialist to assess the needs of your operatory.

Oftentimes it is not the design of ergonomic equipment but the use and adjustment of it that contribute to musculoskeletal problems. These guidelines may help you determine if your operatory layout, design and delivery systems may also be delivering pain.

# CHAPTER EIGHT

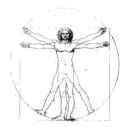

# Managing
# Your Pain

Pain makes man think. Thought makes man wise.
Wisdom makes life endurable.

JOHN PATRICK

A s every dental professional understands, prevention (whether considering dental disease or musculoskeletal conditions) is easier and less costly than treatment. It is my end goal that the research-based information in this book will be used by educators, students and new dentists to prevent musculoskeletal pain largely before it develops and especially before it becomes chronic. As has been shown, however, statistics clearly indicate that a majority of dental practitioners have existing musculoskeletal pain symptoms.

Since you're reading this book, chances are good that you may already be experiencing some occupational pain. Chapters 1 and 2 provided you with a basic understanding of how pain syndromes develop in dentistry. With this knowledge, you are better equipped to take charge of your own musculoskeletal health and make wise choices to manage your own pain.

The pursuit of pain relief can be expensive, time-consuming and frustrating. You may have found that your healthcare provider has little to no understanding of your unique occupational demands and may offer treatment or advice (medication, time off work) that yield only temporary relief.

In this chapter, you will learn strategies for self-managing pain, including determining whether your pain can be self-managed, when it's necessary to call a physician, how to pick the right healthcare provider, developing a recovery schedule and deciding on the most effective therapy.

# Red-Flag Symptoms

First and foremost, it is important to know when you should attempt self-treatment and when you should consult your physician. These are red-flag symptoms that may not be musculoskeletal in origin. If you experience any of the following in conjunction with pain, *call your doctor immediately.*

- If symptoms move frequently from one area to another
- If symptoms *increase* when resting or during the night
- If you cannot reproduce the pain by palpating the affected area, with body movement or positioning
- If the symptoms cover a large, ill-defined area and are hard to pinpoint
- If you have a history of serious illness, especially cancer
- If you experience sudden weight loss or fever
- If you experience numbness or muscle weakness that does not resolve or are unable to bear weight on the lower extremities
- If you experience dizziness, blurred vision, nausea, severe headache, loss of balance or incontinence

You also should see a doctor before initiating any stretching or exercise program if you have had previous surgery, including on your back, neck, shoulders, arms, wrists or hands; if you have had a previous injury that required x-rays, especially a motor vehicle accident; or if you have a pre-existing medical condition, including hyperlordosis, spondylosis, bulging discs, osteoporosis or scoliosis, diabetes or other serious conditions that limit or affect your physical activity.

# Acute Pain

Acute injuries are those with a sudden onset, usually within the time-frame of one day. At some point in your life, you have probably experienced acute pain associated with some type of acute injury. Characteristics of acute pain include:

- Pain at rest (usually severe; a seven or eight on a scale of 10)
- Swelling, redness or heat in the affected area
- Restricted movement in the painful region
- Short duration of only three to five days

Acute injuries can develop into chronic injuries, which are much more difficult to treat and require a longer rehabilitation period. A dental example of this is an acute periodontal abcess vs. chronic periodontal disease. *Hence, early reporting and treatment of musculoskeletal symptoms during the acute stage is extremely important to prevent injuries and or disability.* There are numerous effective treatments that can, if applied early, prevent worsening of symptoms or a trip to the doctor.

# Treatment of Acute Musculoskeletal Pain

You should see a doctor if your symptoms worsen, if they last more than two days, or if you experience any of the previous red flag symptoms.

The acronym "SCRIPT" can help you remember what treatments to try with acute pain:

## *Schedule time for healing*

In an ideal world, team members with acute pain would be able to take two weeks off of work to allow their bodies to heal. Unfortunately, this is not an ideal world. Nevertheless, it is important to consider scaling back your work schedule to allow your body to heal. Schedule either shorter days or days off between workdays, to allow your body's rate of repair to exceed the rate of daily damage (or microtrauma). Don't group your working days (i.e., schedule three 10-hour days in a row followed by four days off).

## *Consider anti-inflammatory drugs*

In the acute phase, swelling can compress surrounding nerves and important structures. Consider medication to prevent edema and to control pain. Consult your physician if you have concerns or have not previously used anti-inflammatory drugs.

## *Rest the area*

Avoid sustained weight on the area, which can aggravate or worsen pain. For example, take the weight off your neck muscles by using armrests or hanging your thumbs in your pockets. Bedrest for short periods may be helpful, but try not to stay in bed longer than 24 hours during this phase.

## *Ice it*

Cold therapy or ice packs are indicated for many acute injuries, including acute muscle spasms, tendonitis, bursitis and sprains. Cold therapy applied early on to the affected area during the acute phase may reduce pain and swelling, and may decrease the chances of a progression to a chronic problem. Carefully follow the guidelines and precautions for heat and cold therapy before attempting hot or cold therapy.

# HOT AND COLD THERAPY

I recommend that every dental office keep a hot/cold pack in the freezer for emergency treatment.

## COLD PACKS

Cold packs are generally indicated for acute pain or injury and are most effective when pain is caused by muscle spasms, inflammation or swelling. Guidelines for use of cold:

- Ice after an initial new injury or flare-up of an old injury.
- At home, use a wet cloth between your skin and a homemade ice pack.
- Ice only until you get a numb feeling, not more than 20 minutes every two hours. Over-icing is not beneficial and can damage tissue.
- Check your skin before, during and after cold application for signs of frostbite. Stop if your skin turns white or hard.
- Use cold after stretching and exercise, if painful.
- Normal sensations during cold application are cold, then ache, then burning, then numbness. Stop usage if pain develops.
- Always consult your doctor before using cold if you have diabetes, circulatory problems, or other underlying health issue.
- Never ice over the front or sides of your neck.

## HOT PACKS

Hot packs are usually the best choice for chronic pain—stiffness and dull achiness that are characteristic of muscular-type pain. Guidelines for use of heat:

- Use a damp towel between a nonelectric hot pack and your skin, since moist heat is more effective than dry heat.
- Do not put heat over topical pain relieving creams.
- Check skin before, during and after heat for rash, blistering or abnormal changes. Stop if skin becomes bright red or blotchy red and white.
- Use heat for up to 20 minutes. Allow one hour between applications.
- Use heat before stretching to relax muscles and to gain the best range of motion from the stretch.
- If heat or ice alone does not help, consider combining the two. Oftentimes, alternating between hot and cold therapies is helpful when transitioning out of the acute phase (after five days or so).

## *Protect and support the area*

Using a wrap, slings, braces, crutches or a cane can accelerate healing by reducing strain on painful areas. Remember that the use of assistive devices during acute or chronic musculoskeletal injuries should be temporary or intermittent. Use of a postural aid is no substitute for strengthening your postural muscles. Make sure you receive proper instruction on using an assistive device, as improper use can result in nerve injury, occlusion of blood flow, skin injury or unsafe ambulation.

## *Treatment by the proper healthcare professional*

(*Note:* If you are considering purchasing disability insurance, it is a good idea to have it in place before you visit a doctor. Disability plans often exclude any areas of the body for which you have sought medical treatment by a physician and are in your permanent medical records.)

Who do you usually turn to when you are in pain? For most of us, it is our primary care medical physicians. Though most physicians have limited training in therapeutic rehabilitation, many are making treatment decisions.

Many dentists encourage their patients to take ownership of their oral health needs and become more involved in treatment decisions. If this is your chairside philosophy, make it a part of your own healthcare needs.

It may be helpful to bring this book to a healthcare professional who understands soft tissue, muscle imbalances and trigger points. This may help bridge the gap of knowledge between your occupational demands and your healthcare professional. Consider requesting a referral to one of the following healthcare professionals for either acute or chronic pain problems.

*Physical therapist (PT).* Physical therapists perform differential tests and evaluations to determine the origin of pain syndromes. They work to regain normal movement and function of the body through use of various modalities, hands-on techniques and exercises. A cornerstone of physical therapist treatment is patient education to prevent re-injury. Most physical therapists have a master's or doctorate degree.

*Occupational therapist (OT)*. Occupational therapists work to restore activities of daily living and occupational skills. They specialize in rehabilitation of the hand and arm and also develop assistive devices to enable workers to return to their jobs. Most OTs have a bachelor's or master's degree.

*Certified hand therapist (CHT)*. A certified hand therapist is an OT or PT who has a minimum of five years of clinical experience, including 4,000 hours or more in direct practice in hand therapy and has passed a comprehensive certification test. If you suspect your problem originates in the hand, wrist or arm, you may want to request a referral to this specialist.

*Certified neuromuscular therapist (CNMT)*. Neuromuscular therapy utilizes specific soft tissue manipulation techniques, flexibility stretching, joint mobilization, neuromuscular re-education, client education and home care to eliminate the causes of most neuromusculoskeletal pain patterns. It is used to locate and release spasms, eliminate trigger points, restore postural alignment and correct biomechanics. Certification for neuromuscular therapy involves an intensive 10-day seminar series and post-test. A CNMT is usually a physical, occupational or massage therapist.

*Osteopathic physician (DO)*. A doctor of osteopathy is licensed to practice medicine and surgery, similar to an MD. However a DO is trained to treat the whole person, not just specific symptoms. They also perform osteopathic manipulative treatment, which may be helpful in relieving certain musculoskeletal disorders. DOs must complete four years of undergraduate study, followed by four years of medical education. They also must complete a residency lasting three to six years following their medical education.

*Chiropractors (DC)*. Based on the theory that disease results from lack of normal nerve function, chiropractors manipulate the spine to realign the vertebrae and relieve pressure on the nerves. Most chiropractic programs require a bachelor's degree followed by 4 years of specialized chiropractic training. CAUTION: *Make sure your chiropractor also addresses any muscle imbalances, or this therapy may not resolve the underlying problems.*

*Pete Egoscue Clinic.* Anecdotally, I have met dental professionals who have benefited from the postural re-education training of Pete Egoscue's clinics. There are many clinics nationwide.

*Surgeons.* While surgery is sometimes necessary, I feel this should be a last resort after all conservative treatment options are exhausted. Although back surgery may be indicated in special instances, studies show that 90 percent of patients undergoing back surgery have returned to work in four years, yet 92 percent have returned to work after conservative, *nonoperative,* treatment.[1] If surgery is recommended, it is wise to get a second opinion and also consult with a therapist who specializes in treating your specific injury before an irreversible procedure is performed.

There are numerous other alternative treatments that may be beneficial as well, such as acupuncture, craniosacral, biofeedback, psychosomatic, hypnosis or cognitive-behavioral therapies.

## MASSAGE THERAPY

A very beneficial therapy for dental professionals is massage. It is effective in the management and prevention of many risk factors known to cause MSDs among dental professionals, including trigger points, emotional stress, muscle spasms, ischemia, and joint contractures, to name a few. Massage may be especially helpful for back pain and may reduce costs of care after an initial course of therapy more effectively than either acupuncture or spinal manipulation.[10]

As with any healthcare professional, the competence of massage therapists depends on the amount of training and continuing education courses they have pursued. Massage therapy school certification programs range from 150 to 2,200 hours of schooling.

## MOVEMENT THERAPY (SOMATICS)

The way you use and hold your body can sometimes lead to a number of pain syndromes. Stress can further aggravate the situation.

Your body responds to stress and postural demands in the operatory with a certain set of habitual, involuntary neuromuscular reflexes. These reflexes can lead to pain and stiffness.

People are creatures of habit. We often find one way of doing something and continue that movement pattern until finally a neck, wrist or back breaks down. You can explore how to re-educate your learned movements to improve your comfort in the operatory through movement exercises developed by Moshe Feldenkrais and Thomas Hanna (founder of the field of Somatics). Another method, the Alexander Technique, focuses on movement, balance and coordination to help students relearn balanced posture and improve movement patterns.

# The Path of Least Resistance

After acute symptoms have resolved and you're feeling "normal" again, it is tempting to discontinue recommended exercises and stretches. This is the biggest mistake you can make. Pain tends to take the path of least resistance, so old injuries are often the first to flare up. Indeed, after an acute injury, your risk for a future flare-up in that area increases dramatically.

You may decrease your frequency of exercising, but stopping completely can toss you right back into the vicious pain/injury cycle or lead to a chronic pain syndrome. (Fig. 1)

Continue stretching and strengthening exercises as recommended by your therapist. Long-term preventive techniques can stabilize your condition, just like your periodontal patients. Remember, avoid any activities or exercises that worsen your pain.

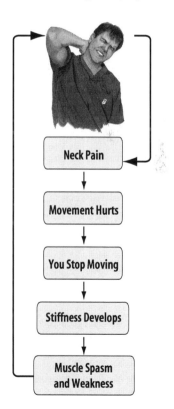

**Fig. 1: The recurring pain cycle. Movement is essential to prevent worsening of symptoms**

Neck Pain
↓
Movement Hurts
↓
You Stop Moving
↓
Stiffness Develops
↓
Muscle Spasm and Weakness

# Chronic Pain

Chronic pain is most common among the dental team, due to years of accumulated microtrauma from numerous risk factors and is characterized by:

- Moderate pain (Ranges 3 to 5 on a scale of 10)
- Localized pain that is felt intermittently, or "off and on"
- Recurring problem

In dentistry, the most common chronic pain syndromes develop due to years of dysfunctional posture and movement. Because the onset is insidious, recovery from chronic pain usually takes longer, and change of habits is required.

Studies on the effectiveness of various pain treatments among dentists and hygienists in the United States found that *permanent* pain relief was obtained by only 16 percent of dentists and 36 percent of hygienists.[2,3] The most effective interventions were as follows (in approximate order of effectiveness):

1. Chiropractic
2. Exercise
3. Reduced weight
4. Different stool
5. Physical therapy
6. Medication
7. Brace/corset
8. Changing positions relative to patient
9. Fewer practice hours

Although pain relief was experienced by a minority of dentists and hygienists in these studies conducted in 1987 and 1990, many advances in equipment technology have developed in the past 20 years. Additionally, much of the research and related prevention strategies in this book were not available at the time of the study.

---

# LOW-BACK PAIN

Low-back pain can be debilitating. Here are a few additional strategies to manage low-back pain:

- Avoid sitting for longer than 20 minutes at a time.

- Lay on your back with your legs elevated on a chair or pillows (hips and knees at 90 degrees), 30 minutes, two to three times a day. This can be done in a patient chair at lunchtime if you are having a flare-up.

- If indicated, perform appropriate chairside stretches and strengthening exercises for the low back.

- Learn to release emotional tension you may be holding in your back muscles. (Chapter 10)

**Tilt table**

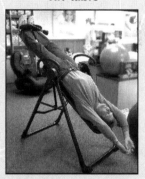

Consider using an inversion table to provide gentle traction to the low back, stretch muscles and renourish spinal discs. This has been a very helpful therapy for many male dentists I have worked with. Always consult your doctor before using an inversion table. Extending over a Swiss ball works similarly, but also places the spine in extension. This helps counter spine dysfunction resulting from chronic forward flexed postures, as in dentistry.

**Swiss ball extension**

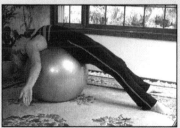

If you experience severe low-back pain (emergency room type), apply ice and lay on your side with a pillow between your legs or on your back with your knees bent and elevated on pillows. See a doctor as soon as possible.

# Steps to Managing Chronic Pain

If your symptoms are not acute, and you have ruled out red flag symptoms, treatment of chronic pain should follow a general sequence:

## 1. Ergonomics in the operatory

First, you should resolve any ergonomic issues in your operatory. This may be done before or concurrent with treatment by a healthcare professional. If not, you may just re-aggravate your injuries when you return to the operatory.

## 2. Pick the right healthcare professional

If you have had persistent chronic pain for longer than six to eight weeks, you should probably consult a healthcare professional.

## 3. Resolve trigger points

Major trigger points should be resolved before any strengthening exercise is attempted.

## 4. Flexibility/range of motion

Chairside and home stretching will help you regain full range of motion and prepare you for strengthening. Overstretching muscles with active trigger points may cause microtearing of muscle. Pain will be your first indicator that the muscle you are stretching may have trigger points. Regardless, you should never stretch in a painful range. Use of heat or whirlpool before stretching helps relax the muscle and increases the effectiveness of the stretch. See Chairside Stretching in Chapter 2.

## 5. Strengthen stabilizing muscles

Studies show that dentists with better endurance of the back and shoulder girdle muscles have less musculoskeletal pain.[4,5] However, if you over-strengthen muscles with trigger points, your pain may worsen. Consider waiting until you are pain-free to begin strengthening.

Allow several weeks to a month to see improvement; your condition took a long time to get this way, so don't expect instant results. Be patient, but most of all commit yourself to a regular regimen of prevention strategies in and out of the operatory. The good news is that you *can* usually treat, manage and prevent chronic pain.

"Working through the pain" may possibly be the single largest contributing factor to pain and injuries in the dental care industry. Time constraints are constantly an issue, so you press on, regardless of the pain. The pain may temporarily go away but usually returns in a worsened state, as is typical with chronic pain conditions. Listen to your body's signals and address any discomfort immediately by using one of the techniques in this book: take a break, change positions, stretch, etc., but do not work through the pain.

# Trigger Points

As described in Chapter 1, painful trigger points are common among dental operators due to several risk factors, including body asymmetry, poor postures, poor body mechanics, repetitive movement, lack of movement, sustained muscle contraction and mental stress.[6] Unfortunately, trigger points are one of the most frequently misunderstood causes of pain and are often the cause of "mysterious" pain syndromes that may be overlooked in traditional Western medicine.

# The Ubiquitous Trigger Point

Trigger points are a common cause of pain in the general population. These painful points can develop suddenly due to whiplash, falls, fractures, dislocation, joint sprains or excessive exercise, or gradually due to muscle overload, poor posture, mental stress and muscle imbalances.[6] Trigger points associated with these events can linger for years afterward if left untreated.

Among dentists and hygienists, trigger points occur in numerous muscles. Two commonly occurring areas are the upper trapezius and lev-

**Fig. 2: Common trigger points and pain referral patterns in dental operators. A.) Upper trapezius, and B.) levator scapulae**

(Travell, Simons, *Myofascial Pain and Dysfunction: The trigger point manual.*
Edited, EP Johnson, Wilkins & Wilkins 1999. Reproduced with permission.)

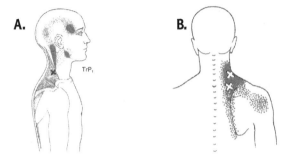

ator scapulae muscles. (Fig. 2) Trigger points in the upper trapezius muscles are a primary source of "tension neckaches." Levator scapulae trigger points can cause pain in the crook of the neck and shoulder. This can lead to stiffness in the neck, making it difficult to look over the shoulder. Although too numerous to cover in entirety in this chapter, other troublesome spots for trigger point development among team members are the scalenes, rhomboids, sternocleidomastoid, infraspinatus, pectoralis, and quadratus lumborum muscles, to name a few. If allowed to persist untreated, some trigger points can cause compression on nerves and contribute to syndromes such as thoracic outlet syndrome or pronator teres syndrome (a carpal tunnel-type pain). Other trigger points, such as those in the suboccipital muscles, can be precipitated by an ergonomic issue, such as forward head posture that leads to tension-type headaches.[7] In the operatory, trigger points can develop from improper positioning, poorly adjusted scopes and a myriad of other ergonomic pitfalls.[8] Specific operatory modifications are, therefore, frequently necessary to avoid recurrences of specific trigger points.

# Treatment of Trigger Points

It is important to relieve trigger points as soon as possible to restore nutrient flow to the muscle, prevent muscle imbalances and prevent compression on nerves.

Various approaches to treating trigger points include:

- Physical therapist trained in trigger point therapy, contract/relax technique or muscle energy technique
- Certified neuromuscular therapist (CNMT)
- Massage therapist trained in trigger point therapy
- Therapist trained in spray and stretch technique
- Physician trained in trigger point injection
- Self-treatment

Although professional treatment is often most effective in treating trigger points, it is difficult to schedule appointments as soon or as frequently as needed. Due to costs, time constraints or convenience, self-treatment is often a more practical and economical consideration. You can treat the pain immediately without waiting for an appointment, paying for the treatment and having to depend on someone else.

# Self-Treatment of Trigger Points

You can learn to effectively self-treat your own trigger points at home or at the office. A very effective combination is trigger point self-massage followed by a sustained stretch of the affected muscle.[9] You may use a tennis ball (or balls) in a tube sock or a smaller hard rubber ball against a wall or on the floor to treat trigger points on the flat of your back and buttocks. However, some of the most problematic trigger points (i.e., upper trapezius and suboccipals) are difficult to treat with this method. Most trigger points can be reached using a self-massage tool. (Fig. 3) Use a trigger point reference book that maps out trigger

**Fig. 3: Self-treatment of trigger points using a self-massage tool**

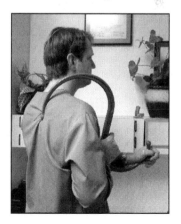

points and the corresponding referral areas to help you easily target your problem areas. (See Resources)

- Locate the trigger point.

- Apply deep pressure for five slow counts, then massage slowly across the point for five counts.

- Alternate between deep pressure and slow massage for *one minute* per trigger point—no longer.

- Aim at a pain level that "hurts so good" (about 5 on a scale of 1 to 10) Don't press too hard on a trigger point, as this can worsen the trigger point *and* your pain.

- Perform a gentle stretch (30 seconds to 60 seconds) to the affected area.

- Treat the trigger point at least three to five times per day, or until pain decreases to a level of one to two on the pain scale. If pain persists longer than two days, or you have any red-flag symptoms, see a physician.

There are multiple strategies that anyone can learn to use to help decrease work-related pain. Your body type, personality, fitness, congenital anomalies and lifestyle are all considerations in determining the best intervention for you.

## SLEEPING POSTURES

Most of us spend about one-third of our lives sleeping, so it makes sense to maintain and support the three primary curves of your spine during that time.

In general, side sleeping can provide you with the most balanced, neutral spinal alignment, if you position yourself correctly. You will need a large, firm pillow under your head that allows you to maintain your head and neck level with the bed. A small pillow or roll between your knees and arms will help reduce low back and intrascapular strain.

Sleeping on your back is all right if you use a very small, thin pillow that does not push your head forward all night long. Also, use a pillow under your knees to reduce compression in the low back.

Avoid stomach sleeping. Sleeping with one arm overhead and your head turned to one side is unhealthy for your neck and shoulder. It is not difficult to retrain yourself from stomach sleeping. Use a contoured neck pillow to support and reinforce your cervical curve at night. These pillows support side and back sleeping but are quite uncomfortable to use in a prone position.

**A contoured neck pillow can help support the cervical curve.**

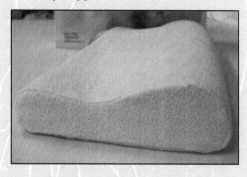

Finally, purchase a mattress that supports your spinal curves. A mattress that is too soft allows the spine to bend, whereas a mattress that is too hard won't support the spinal curves. Newer mattress designs such as adjustable air-filled and memory foam mattresses tend to distribute your weight evenly and reduce compression in one body area.

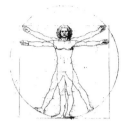

# CHAPTER NINE

# Exercise for
# Dental Professionals

*by Bethany Valachi and Eric Shamus*

---

The doctor of the future will give no medicine,
but instead will interest his patients in the care of the human
frame, in diet, and in the cause and prevention of disease.

---

THOMAS EDISON

No one said you had to be an athlete to be a dental professional, but as clearly described in Chapter 2, the delivery of dental
care is extremely demanding on the body. Physical exercise
has been shown to be an effective preventive intervention for back,
neck and shoulder pain.[1-4] Exercise is especially beneficial for dental
care workers in the prevention and treatment of musculoskeletal disorders and stress[5,6] as well as decreased pain.[7,8] For instance, dentists
with better endurance of the back and shoulder girdle muscles tend
to have less neck, back and shoulder pain.[9,10]

In the quest for the perfect exercise program, you must remember
that your musculoskeletal needs as a dental professional are unique.

You are prone to microtrauma and muscle imbalances that are specific to your profession.[11] Therefore, the *type* of exercise program you embark upon is imperative. The right exercise may prevent injury, improve comfort and increase your career longevity. On the other hand, selecting the wrong exercise can worsen muscle imbalances, increase pain or shorten your career.[12]

So where should you start? First, it is important to understand that there are three components of balanced musculoskeletal health:

- Flexibility (stretching)
- Aerobic fitness (cardiovascular endurance)
- Muscle strength and endurance

As you will see, each of these plays an important role in the prevention of injuries and pain in dental professionals. Remember to always consult your doctor before beginning any new exercise program. Not all exercise is suitable for everyone.

# The Elements of Good Health

## *Flexibility*

Flexibility is the ability of a muscle to relax and stretch to its full length. In the dental profession, prolonged, awkward postures can, over time, cause certain muscles to become short and tight. The asymmetrical shortening of muscles places abnormal strain on the spine and other peripheral joints. This leads to abnormal movement patterns, leading to friction and premature wearing on joint surfaces. For example, if you have rounded shoulders and poor posture the chest muscles (pectoral) will become restricted or tight. The upper back muscles (middle traps, rhomboids) will have to overwork and will tire more quickly trying to overcome the tightness. This is a common postural syndrome (Chapter 4) that creates spasms and pain in the neck, upper trapezius and between the shoulder blades.

Stress can activate the fight-or-flight response (sympathetic nervous system) and result in increased muscular tone. This tightness can result in painful trigger points, muscle spasms or restricted range of motion, which in turn interferes with the performance of many normal daily and leisure activities.

Safe stretching guidelines are described in depth in Chapter 2. The most important flexibility principles are:

- Gentle stretch
- No bouncing
- No pain
- Hold for two to three breath cycles (chairside stretch) or for 20 to 30 seconds or longer if performing stretch at home. Repeat.
- Perform daily

Chairside stretching (Chapter 2) is an important strategy to perform throughout the workday to prevent microtrauma and muscle imbalances. Stretching is especially important after prolonged static postures, and even more so if awkward positions were assumed.

In your home (or gym) exercise routine, you should stretch specific muscles that tend to get tight with prolonged seated operating postures. Certain types of yoga are also excellent ways to develop and maintain flexibility. It is important to warmup *before* vigorous exercise (such as low-level aerobic activity) and to stretch *after* the exercise. Current research suggests that while stretching can decrease pain and soreness after exercise, there is little support for the theory that stretching immediately before or after vigorous exercise can prevent acute injuries.[13]

Your stretching program should include the following muscles:

- Anterior neck musculature (scalenes, sternocleidomastoid)
- Upper trapezius and levator scapulae muscles
- Chest muscles (pectoralis)
- Wrist flexor muscles
- Piriformis
- Hip flexor (iliopsoas)
- Hamstrings

# Aerobic fitness

Aerobic fitness (cardiovascular and pulmonary endurance) is the capacity of the respiratory and circulatory systems to supply oxygen and nutrients to the muscles so that an activity can be performed for a long period of time. To be considered aerobic, an exercise must utilize oxygen to maintain a heart rate for a prolonged period of time through rhythmic and regular joint movement of the large muscle groups. The three primary goals of an aerobic conditioning program are to *improve efficiency of the heart and lungs, develop functional capacity of central circulation* and to *increase blood flow to the working muscles.*

Aerobic activity has been shown to alleviate muscle pain[4] and can prevent musculoskeletal dysfunction and stress for dentists.[9] As stated in Chapter 1, a major contributing factor to MSDs in dentistry is decreased nutrient and oxygen flow to muscles. Aerobic exercise increases blood flow to the tissues of the body, improves their ability to utilize oxygen and improves the body's ability to repair microtrauma. In addition, aerobic exercise may decrease muscle imbalances of the neck and shoulders (Chapter 4) by encouraging use of the primary respiratory muscles while maintaining excellent posture. Diaphragmatic breathing will help relax scalene and anterior neck musculature with aerobic activity. Other main benefits are improvement in cardiovascular and cardiorespiratory function,[14,15] respiratory capacity, lower blood lactate concentration, increased HDL (good) cholesterol, slower resting heart rate, potential reduced cancer risk,[15] decreased blood triglycerides, improved tolerance to stress, increased mental acuity, improved quality of sleep and increased longevity.[15,16] Prolonged, low-level aerobic exercise also helps reduce body fat, an important consideration for dental professionals. Among female dentists, a greater body mass index may be a prescription for low-back pain.[9] Aerobic exercise is also an effective pain intervention for fibromyalgia sufferers; however, this population should avoid impact-loading aerobic exercises like jogging and basketball.

In spite of the popular adage "no pain, no gain," it doesn't take vigorous, intense exercise and sweating bullets to attain good physical fitness. Moderately intense activity such as rapid walking (Fig. 1) while swinging the arms has been shown to have significant health benefits. Rapid walking reduces the risk of cardiovascular disease[14] and may even be even more beneficial than intense physical activity.[15] It is important to remember to wear proper footwear. Certain shoes and sneakers are better for a low arch or high arch. Choosing the correct sneaker may help alleviate low-back pain.

**Fig. 1: Rapid walking while swinging the arms encourages cyclic muscular activitation and may reduce low-back pain**

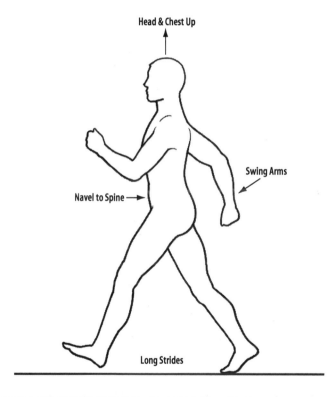

Head & Chest Up

Swing Arms

Navel to Spine →

Long Strides

Walking is the best possible exercise. Habituate yourself to walk very far.
THOMAS JEFFERSON

Due to your predisposition to muscle imbalances, symmetrical-type aerobic exercises are recommended, such as swimming, walking, elliptical trainer (Nordic Track) or cross country skiing. It is advisable to do at least two types of aerobic exercise regularly, for both variety and the benefits of cross-training. You will be much more likely to stick to a program of exercise if you enjoy it and have easy access to it. Be aware of *good posture* with all your exercises. Aerobic exercise should be performed three to four times weekly, or more, for at least 30 minutes.

Certain activities, such as golf, are not considered aerobic since the heart rate is not sustained; a round of golf burns only 300 calories an hour—even when carrying your own clubs. Cart golfers burn roughly the same amount of calories per hour as I did while typing this book!

To safely and effectively participate in an aerobic exercise program, you should first consult your doctor for clearance. To determine the level of aerobic exercise to train at, you need to figure your *target heart rate*.

# Know Your Target Heart Rate

You can find your target heart rate (THR) yourself, or you can purchase a heart-rate monitor at any sporting goods store. First, palpate the radial or carotid pulse for 60 seconds. Your maximum predicted heart rate (MPHR) will be the difference between 220 and your age. For high-intensity exercise (experienced to advanced), your target heart rate will be 85 percent of your MPHR. For low-intensity exercise (beginner), your target heart rate will be 60 percent of your MPHR. For example, if you are 40 years old and your heart rate is 108 beats for one minute while performing the activity, your training level would be 60 percent:

$$220\text{-}40 \text{ (age)} = 180 \text{ MPHR}$$
$$THR = 180 \text{ MPHR X } .60 = 108 \text{ beats/minute}$$

A more accurate method (the Karvonen Method) takes into account your resting heart rate. Use the Karvonen Method calculator online at *www.fitzones.com/members/Fitness/heartrate_zones.asp* to quickly and easily calculate your desired exercise heart rate. Remember, always check with your doctor before beginning any exercise program.

# EXERCISE OPTIONS

### SWISS EXERCISE BALL

The exercise ball has been used in physical therapy clinics in the U.S. for more than 30 years. It is a versatile exercise aid that can effectively address flexibility, core strength, cardiovascular fitness, balance and posture. Working on a Swiss exercise ball is a safe and effective way to target the core stabilizing muscles by creating an unstable base of support from which to move. Numerous stretches may be performed on the ball, which provides a comfortable and firm weight-bearing surface. Perhaps most important among dental professionals, proper posture is facilitated through Swiss ball use, as it promotes a neutral pelvic position. Plus, the ball is a fun and inexpensive way to exercise in your home.

### PILATES

Core strengthening is also the cornerstone of Pilates, a popular exercise regimen that can be performed on a mat or on a specialized machine. This is an excellent program; however, as a dental professional, you should be aware of certain modifications you should make in Pilates programs due to your predisposition to muscle imbalances. A couple of examples include cervical strain or shoulder impingement caused by lifting your head off the mat for prolonged periods or by pushing or pulling overhead against resistance. You may also need to modify or discontinue Pilates exercises that target the upper trapezius muscle. For dental professionals, the safest method to practice Pilates is one-on-one with a physical therapist, certified athletic trainer or doctor who is Pilates-certified and familiar with your unique muscle imbalances. They can weed out the exercises that may cause or worsen pain syndromes.[32] Unfortunately, Pilates certification is not regulated in the United States and requires no background in the health sciences, so use discretion if you are considering any Pilates classes or programs.

### CIRCUIT TRAINING

Circuit training is a method that focuses on muscular strength while utilizing short rest periods. This provides some endurance components while improving muscular strength. The resistance exercises are alternated between body groups to allow for specific muscle recovery while limiting the total body rest time. This allows for more efficiency of time but can limit some of the body mass hypertrophy gains secondary to the decreased recovery times. It is an effective way to improve muscular endurance. The Curves gym is an example of circuit training.

### GYROTONIC EXERCISES

Gyrotonic exercises utilize machines to improve flexibility, balance, joint mobility and muscular strength. The machines simulate movements found in tai chi, swimming, yoga and gymnastics. Anecdotally, I have heard positive feedback from dental professionals regarding this method.

### YOGA

Yoga (meaning "union") is a discipline that engages mind, body and spirit. Through practices of holding a variety of body positions, or asanas, and the centering of the mind and breath in a meditative way, body awareness, posture, flexibility and calmness of spirit are attained.

Hatha yoga is the term used for the actual physical exercises. Several popular types of Hatha Yoga include Iyengar Yoga, by which precise postures are attained through the use of assistive aids; Baptiste Power Vinyasa Yoga, a westernized yoga that teaches intuitive discovery and experiential practices; and Bikram Yoga, practiced in a 110-degree room to encourage perspiration. From a preventive standpoint, yoga is helpful primarily for stress reduction and flexibility.

# Muscle Strength and Endurance

In a society that bombards us with exercise options, from Ab Rollers to ABsliders and Bunbusters, it's hard to imagine that strengthening your muscles could be anything but beneficial. Yet, because of the vulnerability to muscle imbalances, *all strengthening exercise is not necessarily good exercise for dental professionals.* Muscles can be trained for strength, endurance or a combination or both. The selection of training programs will depend on the desired work done by the muscles.

*Muscle strength* is the ability of a muscle to produce force. Increased strength results from recruitment and hypertrophy of Type II muscle fibers (fast twitch). Athletes and those wishing to increase their muscle mass focus on this type of conditioning. Exercise programs to increase strength are characterized by high-resistance, low repetitions and full recovery between each set.[18] Typically, the target of such programs is the "mover or power" muscles, located farther from the center of the body. Examples are the leg and arm muscles, quadriceps, gluteus maximus, latissimus dorsi and pectoralis muscles. Muscle strengthening can create muscle stiffness, so it is important to stretch after each workout.[19]

*Muscle endurance* is the ability of a muscle to repeat a task or hold a contraction over a prolonged period of time without fatiguing. Increased muscular endurance results in recruitment and development of Type I muscle fibers (slow twitch). Exercise programs to improve muscle endurance are characterized by low-resistance, high repetitions and little recovery between sets.[18] Aerobic exercises will also improve muscle endurance. The target of endurance training of the spine is the deep, postural stabilizing muscles, which are closer to the spine. When properly trained, these muscles allow you to maintain an optimal posture for prolonged periods of time without fatiguing. Proper endurance exercise has also been shown to be a protective intervention against low-back pain.[17]

The evidence for selecting endurance exercise over muscle strengthening exercise in dentistry was expressed in a Finnish dental study, "...lack of muscular strength is seldom a critical factor...even among female dentists. While greater muscle strength may protect against overstrain in occupations where greater external forces are frequently applied, it does not seem to protect against symptoms caused by static postural loads."[9]

Studies show that dentists with better endurance of the back and shoulder girdle muscles have less musculoskeletal pain.[20] In dentistry, it is imperative to have proximal stability (excellent endurance of the postural muscles of the trunk and shoulder girdle to stabilize the trunk) so the arms and hands can have distal mobility (perform detailed tasks). When these postural "stabilizer" muscles become fatigued, not only can the operator slump into less than optimal posture, but the "mover" muscles are called upon to perform a stabilizing task for which they are not designed, (i.e., muscle substitution). Muscle imbalances can develop that cause painful trigger points and muscle spasms to develop in the inappropriately used muscle. Also, due to the abnormal muscular tension, joints may not move normally, causing premature degeneration of joint surfaces and inflammation of the muscles or tendons. Over time, weak postural stabilizing muscles in dental professionals may ultimately lead to a CTD. (Fig. 2)

### Fig. 2: Weak postural stabilizing muscles in dental operators may ultimately lead to a CTD

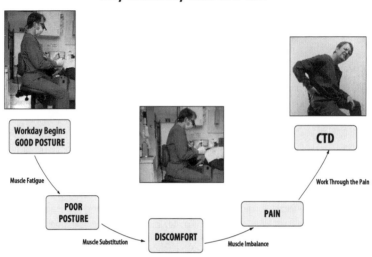

# Balancing Your Muscles

As a result of the vulnerability to muscle imbalances in the shoulder girdle stabilizers (Chapter 4), rotator cuff (Chapter 4) and between the abdominal and low back muscles (Chapter 3), most dentists and hygienists should focus on specific endurance training of the stabilizing muscles of the shoulder and trunk.[12] (Fig. 3-dark shaded) This is especially important for women, who are generally about 50 percent weaker than men in upper body strength and 30 percent weaker in the lower body.[21] In fact, female dentists who have less endurance of the shoulder muscles tend to have more neck and shoulder pain.[10]

Target areas for core endurance training include:[22]

- *Trunk stabilizing muscles:* Transverse and oblique abdominal muscles, quadratus lumborum, erector spinae and multifidus

- *Rotator cuff stabilizers:* Infraspinatus, teres minor, subscapularis and supraspinatus. Care must be taken not to over-strengthen supraspinatus

- *Shoulder girdle stabilizers:* Middle and lower trapezius, serratus anterior, lower rhomboids

Muscles that should be stretched are listed at the beginning of this chapter. This combination of strengthening and stretching addresses a unique pattern of muscle imbalances that can develop among dental professionals.

You should carefully select exercises to avoid over-strengthening muscles already prone to imbalance, tightness, ischemia and pain (Fig. 3-light shaded areas). These include:

- Anterior neck muscles
- Levator scapulae
- Upper trapezius
- Deltoids
- Rectus abdominus
- Pectoralis major and minor

**Fig. 3: Dark shaded – target areas for dental professionals to strengthen: the stabilizing muscles of the trunk and shoulder girdle. Light shaded – areas to avoid over-strengthening that can lead to imbalance, tightness and ischemia**

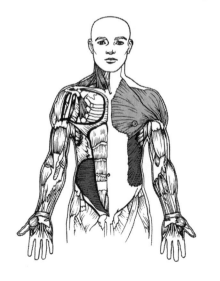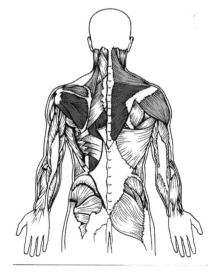

# Guidelines for Endurance Strengthening

Since the postural stabilizing muscles (Fig. 3-dark shaded) perform low-level static contractions for prolonged periods, they must be trained for endurance in a similar manner. These are general guidelines only; each person should be evaluated to determine appropriate exercises in light of their physical condition.

- Use light resistance and high repetitions (15 to 20 reps) when training these muscles. A lightweight elastic exercise band (yellow) works well for the shoulder muscles, while gravity-resisted exercise on the floor or an exercise ball is good for the trunk muscles.

- Begin with the minimum number of repetitions and increase repetitions gradually. You should not increase to two sets until you have performed the exercise for two weeks with no pain.

- Perform endurance exercises three times a week (three sets, 15 to 20 reps), always allowing one day between sessions. Stretches can be performed daily.

- Exercises should be done regularly and should not cause pain. Mild muscular soreness that lingers for an hour or so after you have stopped exercising is normal, but if you experience pain, stop the exercise.

- Stop exercise immediately if you experience numbness, tingling, dizziness or shortness of breath.

- Individuals with carpal tunnel symptoms who work out with weights or on machines should use gloves with wrist straps to lessen compressive forces required to grip handles.

You should begin strengthening exercises only when you have no musculoskeletal pain and full range of motion is present. Consult your doctor when beginning a new exercise, especially if you have a history of injury or illness or if you experience any red flag symptoms. (Chapter 8) It is a good idea to seek guidance from a healthcare professional to ensure good technique.

Following (Figures 4-12) are examples of exercises that target the shoulder girdle, rotator cuff and trunk stabilizing muscles. These types of exercises should be the cornerstone of your exercise program. You may add these to an existing workout routine, or ask your physical therapist, certified athletic trainer or personal trainer for additional exercises that target these areas. Keep in mind that while certified athletic trainers must have a bachelor's degree in athletic training and pass a three-part exam to become certified, personal trainers may not necessarily have certification or a higher education in the health sciences.

Regardless of the avenue you take to get there, be aware of certain exercises that can worsen imbalances and make your muscles miserable. Once you have developed balanced musculoskeletal health through targeting the areas in this chapter, you may wish to progress to a higher level of training. One that is commonly used by athletes is functional training which focuses on dynamic stability exercises with the spine in an upright position (seated or standing).[23]

You will find a complete exercise DVD program developed specifically for dental professionals, *Smart Moves for Dental Professionals On the Ball* at *www.posturedontics.com*. The instruction manual also includes many exercises that can worsen dental professionals' musculoskeletal health. Whatever your age, improving your muscular strength and endurance, flexibility and aerobic fitness will positively impact your susceptibility to injury and your ability to recover.

### Fig. 4: Downward Squeeze

Downward Squeeze targets the shoulder girdle stabilizers. Position door anchor above head level. Loosely wrap band around both hands and position arms at sides, fingers pointing upward. Maintain optimal head posture (ear-over-shoulder) and pull navel to spine, holding this contraction throughout the exercise. Roll shoulders back and down, squeezing shoulder blades downward and together. Pause two counts and slowly return. Repeat 15 to 20 times.

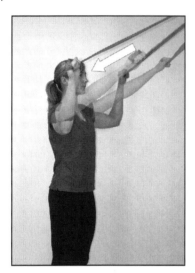 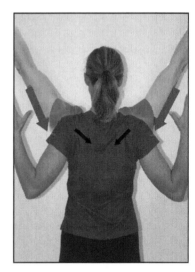

### Fig. 5: Shoulder Rotation

Shoulder Rotation targets the downward gliding muscles of the rotator cuff. Wrap the bands loosely around both hands. Rotate your hands outward, keeping your elbows pressed closely to your side throughout the exercise. Slowly return. The resistance should be easy enough to perform 15 to 20 reps easily. If the resistance is too high, unwrap the band once.

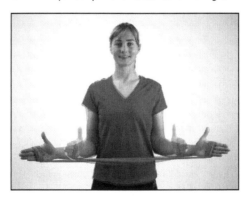

160

## Fig. 6: Side Lift

Side Lift targets the deep trunk stabilizing muscles (transverse abdominal, oblique abdominal and quadratus lumborum).[17] Begin in a side-lying position, and slowly lift both legs off the floor. Hold five seconds. Repeat 5 to 10 times.

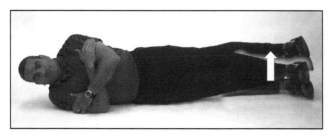

## Fig. 7: Leg Raises

Leg Raises target the transverse abdominal muscles in a supine position. Start with both legs in a bent position. It is important to maintain a neutral, natural curve in the spine. Pull your navel to your spine and hold this contraction throughout the exercise. Slowly extend one leg and lift it off the floor, holding for 5 to 10 seconds. Slowly return and perform on the other leg. Caution: Do not let your back arch off the floor during this exercise. This can damage your low back. If your back arches off the floor, make the exercise easier by lifting your legs higher in the air.

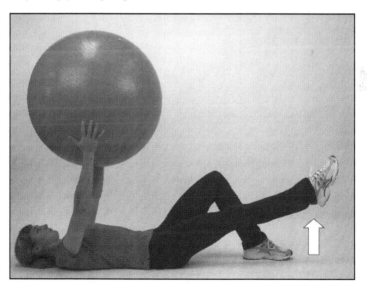

### Fig. 8: Pointer Dog

Pointer Dog strengthens both the trunk and shoulder girdle stabilizers as well as the back and hip extensors.[24] Position yourself on hands and knees and pull your navel up toward the ceiling. Hold this contraction throughout the exercise. Make sure your back is flat and hips are level. Slowly lift the right arm, thumb pointing up, hold for 5 to 10 slow counts and then lower it. Slowly lift the other arm, hold, then lower. Remember to continue breathing. Repeat for each leg. Continue to perform 5 lifts on each arm and leg. Once you master this portion, progress on to the Pointer Dog Challenge: Inhale, exhale lift the right arm and left leg together. Make sure you are still holding your abdominal contraction. Now switch sides. Repeat 15 to 20 times each side.

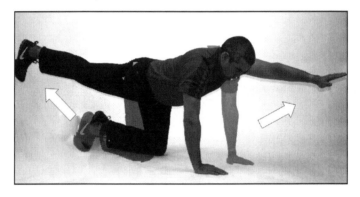

### Fig. 9: Back Extensions

Back Extensions are especially important for dental professionals to increase endurance of the erector spinae muscles, which may prevent low-back pain.[17, 20] Rest your trunk over a ball and clasp your hands lightly behind your head. Slowly raise your head, neck and upper back until your upper body is parallel to the floor. Slowly lower and repeat 15 to 20 times. A roman chair can also be substituted for this exercise. No heavy weights should be used during these extensions, as they place unsafe forces on the spinal discs.[17]

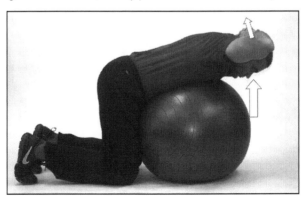

## Fig. 10: Ab Crunches

Ab Crunches target the rectus abdominal and oblique muscles. Lay on your back, with both knees bent. Support the head by placing both hands behind the head, elbows wide. Keep your upper back and neck in a straight line as you slowly lift your chest and chin toward the ceiling, lifting your shoulder blades completely off the floor. Do not let your hands pull your head forward. Hold 2 seconds, and slowly return. Complete 15 to 20 repetitions of this exercise.

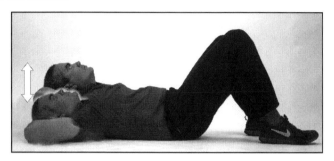

## Fig. 11: Chest Stretch

With elbows at shoulder height, lean into a doorway till you feel a stretch in the chest musculature. Hold 30 seconds, repeat. You may also perform this stretch with hands at shoulder height to target different muscles.

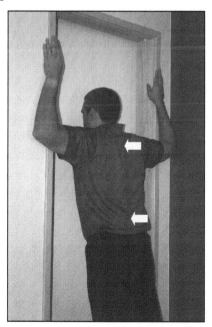

### Fig. 12: Piriformis Stretch

Lying on your back, place your left heel on a ball and position your right ankle across it (left). Gently roll the ball toward you to increase the stretch. A stretch should be felt in the mid-buttock on the right. Hold 30 seconds. Repeat on other side. This can be performed without the ball in the same position by pulling the left knee to your chest while having the right leg crossed over (right).

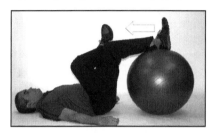 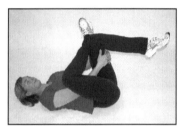

# Golf and Dental Professionals

*Golf and dentists.* We all know they go together like apple pie and Chevrolet. However, the sport that most dentists flock to after work, on weekends or at conferences may make them more susceptible to pain. Among both amateur golfers and dentists, more than half report that the low back is the area most frequently injured.[25] Consider the posture frequently assumed by right-handed dentists and golfers, flexed forward, leaning to the right and rotated to the left. Is it any wonder that both populations experience similar pain syndromes? (Fig. 13)

Addressing two risk factors that contribute to low-back pain in both dentists and golfers may help golfing dental professionals more comfortably continue the sport they love.[26] These risk factors are flexed spinal posture and poor spinal rotation away from the patient, or toward the backswing side. The following exercises and references are for right-handed golfers. Left-handers will need to reverse the directions.

We have seen that *flexed spinal posture* is a common position assumed by many dentists and often difficult to avoid due to varying patient size, poor patient tolerance to reclining, location of the occlusal surface, etc. Flexing the spine forward over the patient is a risk factor for muscle strains, trigger points and disc degeneration or herniation that can result in low-back pain.[11]

## Fig. 13: Dental professionals who golf may be worsening microtrauma that starts in the operatory and leads to low-back pain

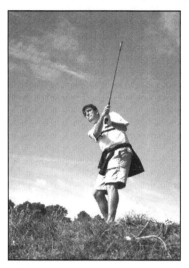 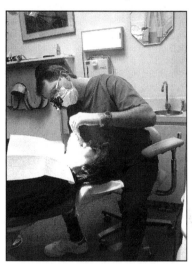

Golfers with low-back pain tend to flex their spines forward when addressing the ball,[27] which tends to limit the amount of spinal rotation. (Fig. 14, left) This may be due to tight hamstrings, habit or poor abdominal strength. Golfers with low-back pain also had significantly less endurance of the deepest abdominal stabilizing muscles, the transversus abdominis, when compared with nonsymptomatic golfers.[28] Poor strength in this muscle will predispose both dentists and golfers to a slouched working posture.

To avoid this damaging posture, dentists and golfers should make it a habit to actively pull the navel to the spine (which activates the transverse abdominal muscle) and pivot forward from the hips, not the waist, whenever leaning forward. (Fig. 14, right)

Engaging the transverse abdominal muscles in this manner helps stabilize and protect the lumbar spine and facilitates proper pivoting at the hips both in the operatory and on the green.[25,29] Not only should the deep abdominal muscles be the target of a strengthening program for dentists and golfers to decrease low-back pain, but also the other trunk stabilizers: quadratus lumborum, lumbar multifidus, erector spinae and oblique muscles. The Swiss exercise ball is one excellent

**Fig. 14: Flexing the spine forward is a risk factor for low back pain (left). Stabilizing with the transverse abdominals and pivoting forward at the hips (right) are important techniques to prevent back pain**

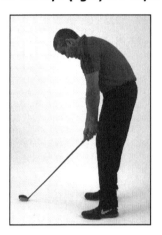 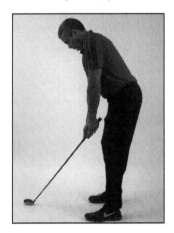

way to target these groups; however, the golfing dentist should also progress to standing exercises that are more functional to the sport.[25]

The second risk factor, *poor spinal rotation*, is also shared by golfers and dentists alike. A certain degree of rotation is difficult for most dentists to avoid in the operatory, and when it occurs, it is usually in one direction. One study showed that right-handed dentists leaned forward to the right and rotated to the left (Fig. 13) for two-thirds of their working hours.[30] Dentists who repeatedly postured this way had the highest incidence of low-back pain and also tend to have less spinal rotation to the right (away from the patient). As we saw in Chapter 3, repeatedly twisting the trunk in one direction (i.e., toward a delivery system or a patient) can also lead to the development of muscle imbalances that cause low-back pain.[31]

Likewise, the body mechanics of right-handed golfers somewhat simulates dentists in the operatory: leaning forward and rotating to the left at the end of their swing. Golfers with low-back pain also tend to have less flexibility with trunk rotation,[27] which can cause compensatory movements in the spine, hips or shoulders.[25]

The golfing dentist should incorporate specific trunk rotation exercises (Fig. 15), especially stretches toward the backswing side (or "away from the patient"), as this is the direction that is most problematic for both populations.[25] Also of importance is avoiding a muscle imbalance of the trunk rotators (oblique abdominals) by targeting the oblique abdominal muscles in a strengthening program.

Anecdotally, I have encountered several dentists who felt they had to quit golf because of their pain. Quitting the sport you love may be unnecessary if these additional exercises and preventive strategies are addressed.

Embarking upon an exercise program requires prudence and discretion, considering dentists' predisposition to certain muscle imbalances. Selecting improper exercises can lead to imbalance, ischemia, nerve impingement and other pain syndromes.

However, when compared with positioning aids, education, ergonomic interventions, and risk factor modification, *proper exercise* has been shown to be the most effective preventive intervention.[2] Developing balanced musculoskeletal health with a well-designed exercise program can help dentists prevent work-related pain, avoid injuries, extend their careers and improve their quality of life.

### Fig. 15: Dental professionals who golf should ensure good trunk flexibility toward their backswing side (or away from the patient)

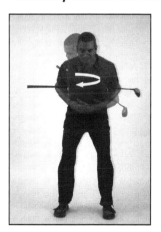 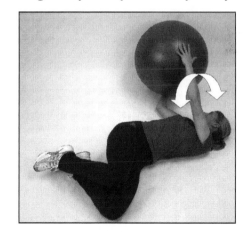

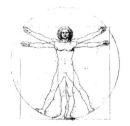

# CHAPTER TEN

# When Dental Goes Mental

The components of anxiety, stress, fear, and anger do not exist independently of you in the world. They simply do not exist in the physical world, even though we talk about them as if they do.

WAYNE DYER

## Stress-Related Pain

The problem of work-related stress in the general population is increasing: from the mid-1980s to the mid-1990s, counseling for work-related stress doubled.[1] In addition, 15 percent of all illness compensation is due to work-related stress.[1]

Common clichés such as "pain in the neck" allude to stress as a cause of pain. This association is actually quite true. Excess tension can elicit muscular contraction and pain, especially in the upper trapezius muscle.[2,3] This type of subconscious muscular contraction in response to stress is called neuromuscular hypertension.[4]

Have you ever noticed that the pain you feel in your neck, back or shoulders coincides with particularly stressful times in your work life?

This is no coincidence. The brain plays a powerful role in muscular tension. As the "electrical powerhouse" of the body, it is responsible for sending electrical impulses to the muscles. With a real or imagined problem, the body produces a "fight-or-flight" reaction. Adrenalin is released, causing an increase in heart rate, blood pressure and respiration and muscular tension to prepare your body to cope with the threatening situation.

In prehistoric times, this fight-or-flight reaction probably saved many of our ancestors from being devoured by toothy predators. However, in the dental office, the fight-or-flight response has little outlet and can manifest itself as muscular tension and, eventually, pain.

Imagine you are a dentist behind schedule on a crown prep for Mrs. Jones. You just dropped into an area of subgingival decay that is deeper than expected. The inflamed tissue starts bleeding profusely, and you must keep reflecting the tissue.

The hygienist rushes in and informs you that while she was treating Mrs. Smith, the veneer on tooth no. 8 just popped off and the patient is very unhappy because she has a job interview in 20 minutes.

It's a situation ripe for stress. But how does your body react? To start with, your muscles fill with tension, preparing for the stressful event. Obviously, you can't flee the office, yet you can't "fight," either ("fight" in the sense that you can't release the building tension).

The stress response then increases heart rate, constricts blood vessels to the visceral organs and expands vessels to the muscles, which raises blood pressure. However, if the stress response is not followed by dynamic muscular activity, the blood pressure has no outlet and continues to rise. The statically contracted muscle becomes ischemic and painful while the blood pressure remains high.[1] This is a common scenario in the dental operatory, where rarely is there a vigorous muscular activity during a psychologically stressful event.

Add to this the Type-A personality common among dental professionals, and the scene is set for psychological mayhem. Dentistry tends to attract Type-A personalities: perfectionists who are ambitious, competitive, impatient and hurried.[5] Compare this to Type-B personalities who tend to be equally motivated and successful but are more able to remain calm and relaxed in stressful situations. Type-A personalities are less tolerant of occupational stress[5] and are at twice the risk for coronary heart disease as Type-Bs.[1]

Stress occurs whenever you to have to adapt to a new situation—the degree of stress that you experience depends on your capacity to cope with those changes. Just as in pain syndromes, there are also two types of stress—acute and chronic. Similar to acute pain, acute stress episodes are generally short in duration, and therefore do not have the time to do the extensive physical damage that results from long-term or chronic stress. In moderate amounts, acute stress can be a good thing. It can stimulate us to a higher level of performance and excellence. On the other hand, chronic stress is more likely to be detrimental to your health.

Like chronic pain, chronic stress develops gradually over a long period of time. Unfortunately, chronic stressors are difficult to avoid. Prolonged and daily stressors—traffic jams that make us late for work, the patient who can't recline all the way, the ortho patient with a severe gag reflex, computer malfunctions—can cumulatively suppress the immune system.[1]

If these daily stressors are mismanaged, they can ultimately lead to psychological afflictions, such as burnout, anxiety and depression.[6] Learning how to manage and prioritize these stressors is key to optimal mental and physical health.

Dentistry is, without a doubt, a very stressful occupation[7,8] and work-related stress can manifest itself as musculoskeletal pain[9] or cause stress-related disorders that lead to early retirement.[10] Dentists themselves rate their occupation as more stressful than other professions,[11] 38 percent of dentists report being "always or frequently worried or anxious."[6]

This stress usually begins in dental school.[12] Drinking is a common coping mechanism among dental students, with 47 percent drinking excessively in their third year and 25 percent in their fourth year. After one year of practice, the number of doctors who drank to excess increased to 41 percent.[13] If not managed correctly, stress can lead to early retirement due to stress-related diseases such as cardiovascular disease (21 percent) and neurotic symptoms (16 percent).[14]

It is difficult to ascertain the degree to which work-related pain causes psychological stress in dentists, or vice-versa; however, studies confirm that dentists with psychological stress experience more musculoskeletal pain.[15]

For instance, dentists with a higher incidence of pain tend to rate their work as "psychologically stressful," have less certainty with regard to their future, less influence over their own work situation, had salary based on commission and a less positive working relationship between their staff and colleagues.[15]

For hygienists, a primary stressor was the presence of musculoskeletal pain, but also balancing work and private life, work organization, long working hours, no assistant, difficult patients, lack of leisure time, lack of support by practice management and doubt about their capabilities.[16]

Smaller dental practices may be less stressful, since job control, support from management and work relations are better, while larger practices may produce more anxiety through increased job demand, poorer control of their job functions, poorer clarity of information from management, more peer pressure and social skill demands.[17]

# What's the Source of Your Stress?

People react to identical stressors differently. The lack of strict patient scheduling guidelines may stress one team member but have little effect on another.

To get your stress under control, begin by identifying your occupational stressors and preventive strategies. Following are some of the most stressful situations affecting dentists and hygienists.

## *Time management*

Running behind schedule is a frequently reported problem by dentists.[8,13,18] Allowing appropriate space for emergency patients can avoid scheduling emergency patients during lunch. Unexpected developments that occur while operating that require a longer, different procedure should be rescheduled.[19] A good practice management consultant can not only help with time management but also can provide skills for dealing with other common stressors, including communication among the team, dealing effectively with anxious or uncooperative patients and insurance billing issues.

## Anxious patients

Anxious patients can be difficult stressors to manage in the operatory.[8] The patient's trust and relationship can be improved by carefully taking thorough histories and encouraging patients to ask questions and express their concerns related to treatment, their unique needs and fears.[5]

## Uncooperative patients

Patients who are chronically late, cancel appointments or do not comply with the practitioner's instructions can be enormously stressful. Fidgety or fearful children also can be a source of anxiety for the dentist and hygienist.[20] It may be in your best interest to limit treatment time for these patients to as short as is clinically appropriate.[5]

## Technical perfection

The constant striving toward perfection and the disappointment of not always achieving it may be more common in Type-A personalities. The ability to be OK with treatment outcomes that are less than perfect but still clinically acceptable is an important coping skill for dental professionals.

## Heavy-calculus patients

Scheduling of consecutive heavy calculus patients can be both physically and emotionally stressful for hygienists.

## Team member controls

Most dentists say that positive interaction with their colleagues and team members contribute to their mental well-being at work. It is important for team members, especially men, to discuss the sources of their stress with each other. Men may tend to hold in their feelings, rather than discuss them openly, and therefore have a far greater risk of developing cardiovascular disease than women. Talking openly about work-related stress at team meetings can lead to the development of realistic, applicable goals that can improve team interaction and reduce stress.[5]

## Job control and dissatisfaction

It is important for good health that staff members perceive their work as meaningful and also have the ability to influence or control their jobs.[15,21] People who feel they have no control have poorer health. This is especially damaging to people who try to control uncontrollable situations.[1]

Hygienists who have more decision-making power in their jobs tend to have fewer musculoskeletal complaints.[21] Most hygienists, however, are less able to influence their jobs than dentists. Improving hygiene skills through continuing education opportunities was also shown to improve job satisfaction.[22] Therefore, it is important that hygienist's job descriptions, CE opportunities, etc., are clearly defined before employment.

Dentists need to feel their work is stimulating and interesting. A lack of intellectual challenge is one cause of job dissatisfaction among dentists. Specialists express greater job satisfaction overall than general dentists.[15] It also was found that stress is lessened in dentists who instruct other professionals.[23]

If none of these strategies seem to work, you may very well be a round peg in a square hole. Perhaps you are simply unhappy in your work environment. You may be in an office where you don't feel like you fit in, or maybe someone in your dental team is a mismatch. Regardless, the solution is obvious—move or get another job.

## Heavy workloads

Arduous work loads[11] and long hours are not only emotionally stressful but are physically taxing as well. To be effective at work, your mind and body need periodic reprieves from work in the form of rest, leisure activities, vacations or recreational sports. If your work is so demanding that you have no time for leisure activities or vacations, you need to re-assess your priorities and consider time for planning a vacation.

# Internal Coping Strategies

Since not all occupational stressors can be completely eliminated, it is important that operators have internal coping strategies to defray the cumulative mental and physical damaging effects of stress. Many dentists use a variety of coping strategies to deal with their stress; however, about 25 percent do nothing.[8] Dentists who report having "personal harmony" have less occupational pain[15] and may have better coping mechanisms to deal with stress.

Given the statistics, this is another area that could be addressed in dental/hygiene schools. All operators should learn techniques to decrease stress-related muscular tension, including breathing techniques, progressive relaxation, visualization, autogenics and exercise.

## *Breathing techniques*

Breathing is easy, right? You've been doing it your whole life. However, improper breathing can contribute to panic attacks, anxiety, depression, muscle imbalances, tension headaches and fatigue.[24]

*Chest breathing* is a shallow type of breathing associated with anxiety and stress. It is frequently unwittingly used in the operatory during procedures. During chest breathing, the chest expands outward and the shoulders rise upward to take in air. The anterior neck muscles also assist with this type of breathing and can become shorter and tighter, especially among dental professionals who are already prone to this muscle imbalance. (Chapter 4) Since chest breathing is shallow, less oxygen is taken in, which can trigger your stress response as your muscles become tense and deprived of oxygen.

On the other hand, *abdominal (or diaphragmatic) breathing* is a more natural type of breathing. This is the way that babies breathe. You do it when you sleep. The diaphragm is actively used to draw air deeply in and out of the lungs, hence your body receives more oxygen. This type of breathing, when done slowly and regularly can elicit a relaxation response of the central nervous system. You can learn to do this by placing one hand over your stomach. Breathe in deeply, as if you were inflating a ball deep in your abdomen. You should feel your hand being pushed outward by the expansion of your stomach. Deep breathing relaxation exercises are easily and discreetly performed chairside, often without your patient's or colleague's awareness.

## Progressive relaxation

It is common in dentistry to subconsciously hold muscles in a contracted state—especially the neck and shoulder muscles. Progressive relaxation allows you to identify and quickly relax tense muscles. This is especially important in the upper trapezius muscle, which is particularly susceptible to emotional stress. Relaxation techniques have been shown to increase the number of natural killer cells in the body, thereby boosting immune function, and also help locate and distinguish between tense and relaxed muscles.

Practice is usually done through a guided audio CD, which takes you through the entire body, alternately tensing the muscle in a particular area for a few seconds, then allowing the muscle to relax. Eventually, you will learn to effectively detect where you are holding muscular tension in your body and quickly release it.

## Visualization

If you have a good imagination, visualization may be a good relaxation tool for you. This is based on the idea that "you are what you think" or more simply put, if you think of happy, relaxing scenarios, you will become happy and relaxed. Once again, it uses guided audio to create in your mind a "happy place," which may be a forest, a beach or a meadow. You may integrate numerous senses to the narration (touch, taste, smell, etc.) to make the experience more effective.

## *Autogenics*

Created by a German neurologist, autogenics creates powerful physiological sensations to verbal suggestions by involving the neuromuscular, vasomotor, cardiovascular and respiratory systems.[4] By repeating a phrase—for instance, "my left arm is heavy and warm" —blood flow is actually increased to that area and relaxation is facilitated in the muscles.

---

### QUICK TENSION BUSTER

This relaxation exercise incorporates four of the most effective techniques for reducing musculoskeletal pain resulting from stress: breathing, progressive relaxation, visualization and autogenics. You can modify the length of this exercise by extending or shortening any of these four components.

Breathe in as you tense fists, bring shoulders up to ears, arch back and extend backward. Exhale, placing one hand on the abdomen, take deep abdominal breaths through your nose and exhale slowly through pursed lips. Close your eyes and release tension in the shoulders, neck, arms and back.

Imagine yourself covered in warm sand at a beach—you hear the waves crashing and seagulls calling overhead. As you continue with abdominal breathing, say the word "warm" as you inhale and "heavy" as you exhale.

---

## *Exercise*

Daily exercise, such as walks, stretching, yoga or resistance training can reduce anxiety and depression and makes people feel more positive and "in control."[1] Aerobic exercise is especially beneficial for "burning off stress," as it reduces the cardiovascular and hormonal reactions that result from psychological stress.[1]

Yoga is beneficial both from a psychological and physical standpoint. (Chapter 9) It helps maintain flexibility in the body by moving through a series of postures combined with deep breathing. This combination of deep breathing and stretching create a relaxation response in the central nervous system. Through regular practice, yoga practitioners report attaining lightness, relaxation, and a sense of peacefulness.

Exercise balls are not only helpful in developing good endurance of the core muscles and treating chronic back pain, but also help relieve stress. Dr. Corey Gould of Neck and Back Medical Center in Laguna Hills, Calif., says that the ball is a fun and inexpensive way to de-stress at home.[25]

## Relaxation stretches

Remember to begin all your daily chairside stretches at work with a slow, deep breath in, then exhale as you stretch to encourage relaxation. (Chapter 2) Every time you stretch, you can make it a relaxation technique by breathing properly. Remember that stretching encourages relaxation of the nervous system. Move in slow, rhythmic movements.

## Massage

Therapeutic massage has been shown to be beneficial in reducing psychological stress.[26] Massage reduces activity of the body's sympathetic nervous system (the fight-or-flight stress response), and increases activity of the parasympathetic system (slowing the heart and respiration, and increasing blood flow to the visceral organs). It also reduces muscle tension and trigger point formation, improves circulation, speeds healing, and has beneficial effects on the skin texture, lymph system, fascia, visceral organs and sweat glands, among many others. The most common type of massage is Swedish massage, which uses a combination of stroking, kneading, rubbing, tapping, vibration and compression to achieve the desired result. Deep tissue and sports massage incorporate firmer, deeper pressure to target specific muscle groups. For both the physical and psychological benefits, I highly recommend regular massage for all team members, one to two times monthly. On site seated massage is becoming increasingly popular and can be a good option for fitting a massage into a tight work schedule.

## *Meditation*

Meditation can also help defray the damaging effects of stress by shifting your focus away from your stressors and putting your mind in "neutral." Many types of meditation are available, some with a religious orientation, others for healing, stress relief or personal achievement. Meditation may be verbally guided, as with a CD, or simply carried out in a quiet setting alone.

Other alternative therapies that may be beneficial in reducing stress are aromatherapy, Bach flower remedies, hypnotherapy, reflexology and Reiki.[27] Don't overlook the importance of the everyday basics in controlling stress: getting the right amount of sleep (at least seven to eight hours), eating properly, a hot bath and drinking plenty of water.

# Mind Over Matter

Glass half empty or half full? You have undoubtedly heard the phrase, "Where the mind goes, the body will follow." This was demonstrated in a study that tracked participants over 30 years and found that pessimists were more prone to illness and died earlier than optimists. Pessimism in early adulthood is a risk factor for poor health in middle and late adulthood.[28] Your mind is like a movie projector, constantly playing scenes and projecting outcomes; however, many people lose sight of the fact that *you* write your own script. Refocusing your thoughts on positive aspects can positively influence your comfort and health.

In Chapter 8, I wrote about "temporary fixes" for pain management. Therapies aimed at immediate relief usually yield temporary results. To this same end, Dr. Wayne Dyer, internationally renowned author and speaker in the field of self-development, offers prudent advice: "Infinite patience yields immediate results." At first this statement confused me. I thought, "That's crazy, because if I wait, it isn't happening right now." Then I realized that my impatience in getting this book done was causing headaches and neck pain. What difference will it make if the book is two months past my arbitrary deadline? None. By being patient with my book deadline, I got immediate results: my neck pain and headaches immediately resolved.

Realize that your life is 1 percent what happens to you and 99 percent how you react. You can choose to allow an event to cause you stress or not. Stress is not something that passively washes over us, but something we make a conscious decision about. It is a result of how we react to our changing situations in life. Simply by realizing this fact, you may alter the way you perceive the world and change your vulnerability to stress.

Ironically, as I approached completion of the writing of this chapter on stress, my computer crashed, and I lost a portion of the chapter. I immediately went into my normal stress mode, realizing the multiple hours and text were lost forever somewhere in cyberspace. I felt my throat constrict and wanted to smash my computer with a hammer (did I mention I hate computers?). Then I realized something that has taken far too long to reach my consciousness. Usually when things like this happen to me, something good comes from it. Looking for the silver lining as I trudged back through my research, I found two segments of research I had overlooked that were critical for this chapter. Looking for the positive instead of focusing on the negative can make life much more pleasurable.

Stressful events are an inevitable part of delivering dental care, but *how* stress impacts your health is up to you. Similar to work-related pain, you can make conscious decisions and take pre-emptive actions to defray the damaging effects of stress in your daily life.

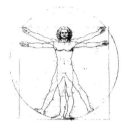

# CHAPTER ELEVEN

*– Bonus –*

# The Dental Assistant

## The Great Accommodator

I magine being in the passenger seat of a car and trying to see over the edge of a cliff to the bottom of a deep canyon. This posture gives you an idea of the ergonomic challenges encountered by dental assistants—significantly different from dentists and hygienists. Assistants are unable to position their knees under the patient, often must twist, cannot freely reposition their chair to different "clock" positions, and must usually accommodate to the dentist's positioning. Combined with poor operatory layout or delivery systems, it is understandable why assistants report that their highest prevalence of musculoskeletal pain is in the low back.[1,2]

A healthy and well-trained assistant can easily boost a practice's productivity and also decrease stress for the dentist. Any dentist who has had a trusted, long-term assistant miss work or leave the practice knows this well. An excellent assistant requires an investment of training on the part of the dentist, which takes time, money and, usually, some stress. The well-trained assistant is, therefore, a valuable asset to the team and should not be viewed as a "disposable" member that can be cheaply replaced if body parts begin to fail. An enlightening exercise for dentists to gain insight to the aches and pains of their assistant is to trade places with them for 20 minutes. The positioning challenges become apparent immediately.

Investment in proper ergonomic training and equipment for the dental assistant can yield large benefits for the team's productivity as well as the assistant's job satisfaction and career longevity.[3]

# CTDs in Dental Assisting

The most common CTD among assistants is chronic low-back pain.[1,2] Other common areas of pain are the neck, shoulders (right more than left), legs, arms and hands. If ignored, this pain may result in muscle imbalances, ischemia, nerve compression or disc degeneration.

To maintain optimal musculoskeletal health, assistants must understand the unique muscle imbalances to which they are prone and how various working postures, positions, adjustment of ergonomic equipment and exercise can positively or negatively affect their musculoskeletal health.

# Posture and Movement

Primary operating tasks of the assistant include keeping the mirror clear, retracting soft tissue, rinsing and drying the field, instrument and handpiece transfers and light adjustment. To gain direct viewing of the oral cavity, assistants often cannot maintain ideal neutral posture, which is ear, shoulder and hips vertically aligned. Viewed from the back, posture of the neutral spine is straight. The upper arms should abduct out to the sides no more than 20 degrees and reach forward a maximum of 25 degrees.[4] The shoulders should be relaxed, not elevated. Assistants should avoid reaching across their midline with the right arm and hand. This can be achieved with proper assistant positioning. Wrists should be as straight as possible when holding suction devices, neither flexed nor extended. The more the body deviates from these neutral postures, the more strain is placed on muscles, tendons, ligaments, joints and spinal discs.

Frequent forward and side-leaning postures to one side are a potent combination and help explain the assistant's increased risk for low-back pain.[5,6] But the assistant also faces the challenge of not being able to easily change chair positions around the patient. Therefore, assistants should seize every opportunity to change their posture and move, either by standing or chairside stretching. (Fig. 1) This is imperative to the assistant's musculoskeletal health.

### Fig. 1: Two primary working postures for the dental assistant: seated and standing

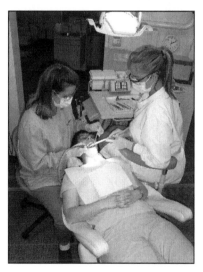 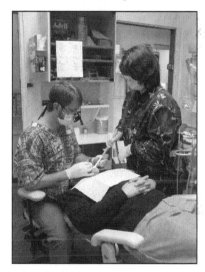

# The Seated Assistant

An area of great controversy for the assistant is use of the dental assisting stool. Specially designed assistant stools have been around for a long time. The unique features of these stools are supposed to increase comfort and help support assistants while they work. The stool should help stabilize the assistant without impairing movement or inhibiting access to the patient. The variety of features can make the selection process confusing.

PRACTICE DENTISTRY PAIN-FREE

Dental assisting stools vary in design: those with backrests only or torso support bars only, and those that have both backrest and a torso support bar. Seat pans vary in size and some even tilt to one side. It is probably due to the variety of assistant stools and positioning challenges that such a wide array of seated postures are observed among assistants. Unfortunately, many of these postures contribute to CTDs.

Important features of the assistant stools with *support bar* include:[7]

- Height adjustment of chair
- Foot ring with adjustable height
- Single torso support bar that ratchets or pivots toward center of seat pan
- Easy, quick adjustment of torso support bar height (no screws)

**Fig. 2: Proper adjustment of the chair and torso support bar promote neutral operating posture**

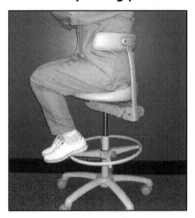

The torso support bar should adjust inward toward the side of the assistant for optimal trunk support. (Fig. 2) This inward adjustment is achieved with either a ratcheting torso support bar or one that pivots inward. Torso bar designs that swing in a circle around the edge of the stool cannot be adjusted inward to provide proper trunk support at the side of smaller assistants. This forces assistants to sit on the edge of their seat to utilize the support bar.[7] Larger-framed assistants may not need this inward adjustment, as the support bars located at the periphery of the stool may already contact their torsos.

Important features of the assistant stools with *backrest only* include:[7]

- Height adjustment of chair
- Foot ring with adjustable height
- Backrest that adjusts up, down, forward and backward

**Fig. 3: Two assistant stool designs:
the single torso-support bar and the backrest-only**

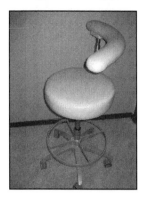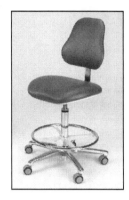

# Stool Adjustment

Assistants of varying heights and sizes will often use the same stool. In such cases, ease of adjustment should be a priority in the selection process. Torso-support bar, foot ring, and/or backrest may need to be adjusted each time a different assistant uses it. A backrest-only design may eliminate readjustment of the torso bar; however, the backrest height may still need to be adjusted.

## *Adjustment for stools with a single support bar*

- Sit all the way back on the seat.
- Adjust the foot ring of the stool up or down so the thighs are parallel to the floor or sloping slightly downward.
- Adjust the height of the torso support bar to just below the bottom rib.

Adjust the torso support bar inward toward the side of the assistant to fit snugly against the torso under the ribs. The end of the bar should be only slightly in front of midline of the torso and provide enough bar support behind the assistant to rest the back. (Fig. 2) This enables the assistant to periodically relax on the support bar to allow the low back muscles to rest and be replenished with oxygen and blood flow.

- Adjust the height of the chair so assistant's eye level is four inches to six inches above the dentist's eye level.

## Adjustment for stools with a backrest only

- Adjust the lumbar support up or down to nestle into the low back curve.
- Once the backrest is adjusted to proper height, angle the backrest *away* from you.
- Sit all the way back on the seat.
- Adjust the foot ring up or down until the thighs are parallel to the floor or sloping very slightly downward.
- Sit tall and angle the backrest of the stool forward to snugly support the low back.

Assistants may need to raise the stool slightly higher with treatment of the lower arch. Shorter assistants working with tall doctors may find their stool will not adjust high enough. If the cylinder won't raise high enough, consider purchasing a different model. Unlike operator stools, which are frequently available in multiple cylinder heights, manufacturers typically offer only one height cylinder for their assistant stool; however, this height varies widely among manufacturers, ranging from about 27 inches to 33 inches. A listing of heights of various manufacturers' assistant stools is available at www.posturedontics.com, under "Product Reviews."

Stools with both a backrest and wraparound abdominal support bar typically do not adjust inward toward the assistant's left side to provide trunk stabilization. (Fig. 4) This may cause the user to face the patient and slump forward over the bar, bending the spine into a "C" shape.

Even with the best chair and adjustments, assistants will intermittently have to leave their optimal posture to gain direct view of the treatment area. Whenever posture deviates from neutral, the dental assistant should practice the Dental Operator Pivot to stabilize and protect the back. (Chapter 3)

Both designs, the single torso-support bar model and the backrest-only model (Fig. 3) allow for easy performance of the Operator Pivot. This exercise helps stabilize and protect the low back when the assistant must periodically lean forward to gain better visibility into the oral cavity.

**Fig. 4: Placement of a bar across the abdomen while squarely facing the patient encourages rounded back posture**

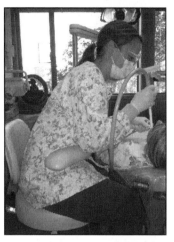

## Seated Assistant Positioning

To maintain neutral posture, the assistant must be seated close enough to the oral cavity to avoid forward leaning. Ideally, the assistant should be seated with left hip at the patient's left shoulder and knees angled toward the patient's head. Most patient chairs are tapered toward the head of the chair and facilitate this position. Thighs parallel with the long axis of the patient is not recommended, as this obviously requires more twisting of the assistant's trunk.

Close positioning may cause the assistant's and doctor's knees to make contact when the dentist is in the 11 o'clock or 12 o'clock position, especially if the dentist or assistant is long-legged. In certain cases, interlocking knees may enable both the dentist and assistant to maintain better positioning during procedures. (Fig. 5) Some dentists and assistants may be uncomfortable with this amount of contact. Overcoming this hesitancy requires professionalism and communication between the dentist and assistant regarding the goal of this positioning, which is to preserve the health of the assistant and deliver quality patient care.

Several other doctor/assistant treatment positions are possible, and some may enable better ergonomic positioning than others. (See sidebar, Pg. 188) The dentist and assistant should evaluate each for its appropriateness for them, considering delivery system, procedure type, operator height and patient chair type.

## Fig. 5: Leg overlap positioning of the assistant with the dentist

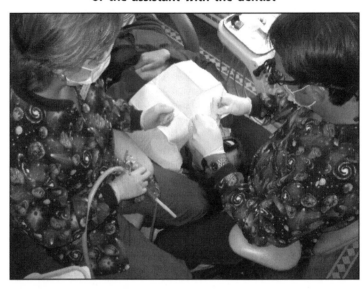

## Doctor & Assistant Treatment Positions

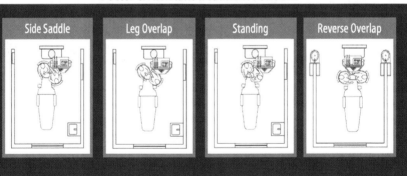

Side Saddle | Leg Overlap | Standing | Reverse Overlap

**PROS:**
- Easy to enter and exit procedures
- Allows class IV & V motion ("pinwheel")
- Doctor operates from familiar position
- Provides wide range of operator motion

**CONS:**
- The least efficient four-handed positioning
- Ergonomically challenging for assistants
- Generally requires belly bar use

**PROS:**
- Brings assistant much closer to treatment field
- Allows greater assistant treatment acuity
- Doctor operates from familiar position

**CONS:**
- Slower entry and exit during procedure

**PROS:**
- Easy to enter and exit procedures
- Allows class IV & V motion ("pinwheel")
- Provides wide range of operator motion
- May alleviate doctor and assistant height mismatch

**CONS:**
- Tiring during long procedures
- May create doctor and assistant height mismatch

**PROS:**
- Brings assistant much closer to treatment field
- Allows greater assistant treatment acuity
- Excellent for lower arch treatment

**CONS:**
- Slower entry and exit during procedure
- Doctor operates best from 7-10 o'clock zone

DESIGN ERGONOMICS
-- www.design-ergonomics.com
Copyright © 2005

# The Standing Assistant

As mentioned previously, the assistant is less able to move around the head of the patient and is most vulnerable to the damaging effects of prolonged, static postures. Assistants should therefore try to stand for up to half of treatment time. Alternating between standing and sitting moves the workload from one group of low-back muscles to another and may help reduce low-back pain.[8,9]

Keep in mind that the assistant should still be four inches to six inches above the dentist's height— even when standing. Certain height combinations will work better for this than others. A medium-height or tall dentist and shorter assistant is the most ideal, since the assistant won't have to bend over while standing. If the dentist is too tall, the assistant can stand on a short platform. (Fig. 6)

**Fig. 6: When standing, the assistant may use a short platform to raise their height**

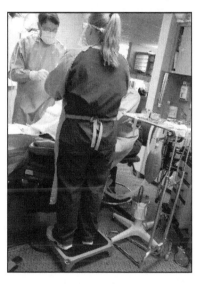

Perhaps the worst combination for standing is a short dentist and tall assistant. One way to make this work from an ergonomic standpoint is for both the dentist and assistant to stand. The assistant should still remember to perform the dental operator pivot in standing (pivoting at the hips) whenever leaving a neutral upright posture is necessary. Again, effective communication between dentist and assistant can help each attain better posture and positioning.

# Assistant Delivery Systems

The assistant's handpieces and instrument tray must be in close proximity. The instrument tray is best positioned directly in front of the assistant, preferably extending over the assistant's lap. Positioning too far away will result in repeated extended reaching or forward leaning. All handpieces and instruments should ideally be within fingertip's reach when the arm is comfortably extended, without leaning.

One type of assistant delivery is on a fixed counter at the 1 o'clock position. These are frequently located too far away from the assistant and cause excessive reaching. If instruments are out of comfortable reach, try swiveling the patient chair 10 degrees to 20 degrees counter-clockwise. This may place the assistant closer to the delivery system.[3] A better solution when utilizing a fixed counter, it is to mount the assistant's work surface on a swiveling tray on a long arm that swings out in front of the assistant, over the knees. Over-the-patient delivery systems should be placed as high on the patient (close to the head) as possible, to discourage backward twisting of the assistant to retrieve handpieces.

Another type of delivery is a mobile cart (a unit on wheels) that can move freely in the operatory. Mobile units are often an effective, inexpensive modification for certain operatories; however, there must be adequate room so the assistant's position is not compromised. Mobile carts often solve positioning problems, as they can be moved to the desired position in the operatory. Assistants should be able to position their knees easily under their delivery system.

# Additional Considerations

The shape of the patient chair can also impact the assistant's posture. Wide "wings" on a patient chair prohibit the assistant from positioning the stool close to the patient, causing side-leaning. (Fig. 7) Note that when the assistant's torso support bar is positioned correctly, the vertical post of the torso support bar does not contact the patient chair.[7]

Because hand and wrist discomfort is common among assistants, they should alternate between palm and pen grasps to avoid overworking one area of the hand and wrist.[7] Gloves should be fit loosely across the palm and around the wrist, and snug in the fingers. This may be difficult for some to achieve with ambidextrous gloves. In this

**Fig. 7: Wide wings on patient chairs prevent close positioning to the patient and cause side-leaning of the assistant**

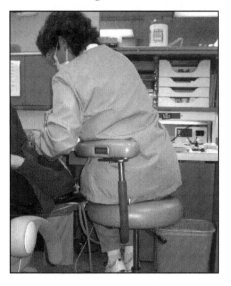

case, fitted gloves may provide a better fit. Hoses on handpieces should also be long enough so excessive force is not necessary while working. If these strategies do not resolve the problem, follow guidelines in Chapter 5. Assistants should consider the possibility of pronator teres syndrome as a cause of hand and wrist pain.[10,11]

Lighting can also impact the assistant's posture. For efficiency, the assistant should adjust the lighting for the dentist. If the light is difficult to pull along a track or to adjust, contact the manufacturer. Repetitive overhead pulling on a stiff light can lead to shoulder problems.[3]

The assistant's position is largely impacted by their view of the oral cavity. For instance, the position of the dentist's fingers on the mirror can force the assistant to assume an unbalanced posture to gain view of the oral cavity. Simply moving the dentist's fingers up or down on the mirror handle can help the assistant's view and posture. Asking the assistant, "Can you see?" before the procedure can go a long way in improving assistant's comfort and career longevity.[7] Communication is key to optimal assistant positioning.

# Exercise

Due to their susceptibility to low-back injuries, assistants should maintain excellent endurance of the trunk stabilizing muscles, especially the transverse and oblique abdominal muscles. (Chapter 9) As with all exercise, always consult your physician before beginning any strengthening or stretching programs.

The assistant is subjected to similar microtrauma resulting from prolonged, static postures and non-neutral postures, as are the dentist and hygienist. For this reason, the assistant should also regularly perform chairside stretches that reverse potentially harmful postures (i.e., primarily away from the patient). Stretches that target the low back are especially important for assistants; however, neck, shoulder and hand/wrist stretches are also important. It is important to know how to stretch safely. (Chapter 2)

Your practice's assistants face unique musculoskeletal challenges during treatment. Using equipment properly, paying attention to proper positioning, and learning about balanced musculoskeletal health all contribute to preventing pain and injuries in dental assisting. Prevention of muscular pain can make the difference between a satisfying, lengthy career in dental assisting or painful early retirement.

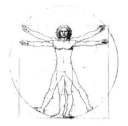

## – *Bonus* –

# "Ergonomizing" Your Front Office

With increasing awareness of ergonomic challenges in the dental operatory, it is easy to overlook ergonomic issues in the front office. Surprisingly, though, the frequency and severity of ergonomic problems in the front office frequently rival those in the operatories.[1]

From an ergonomic perspective, office workers have a slight advantage over their colleagues in the operatory. Office work does not encourage frequent forward leaning or tilting the head down to view their work to the degree of dental procedures. Unlike the dentist and hygienist, with the proper ergonomic workspace, front office workers may actually attain ideal working posture (ear over shoulder over hip). This may be why less attention and lower priority is often given to proper position and equipment for front office workers in dental offices. Unfortunately, this neglect can result in a myriad of musculoskeletal problems and injuries for the front office executive.

As in the operatory, solving ergonomic issues in the front office involves attention to posture, movement patterns and equipment.

However, unlike dental equipment, front office equipment is usually less expensive and, therefore, usually a cheaper fix.

# CTDs in the Front Office

Just as in clinical dentistry, microtrauma (Chapter 1) can occur in the front office on a day-to-day basis without the individual being aware of a problem until the cumulative damage results in pain. Although front office workers are prone to pain in several areas of the body, the 'hot spots' tend to be the neck, shoulders, hands and wrists.[2] Although carpal tunnel syndrome is a frequent complaint among front office executives, this dysfunction is frequently misdiagnosed and often due to nerve irritation in the arm, shoulder or neck, due to poor working posture.[3]

# Front Office Posture

**Fig. 1: Positioning for dental front office workers includes consideration of multitasking**

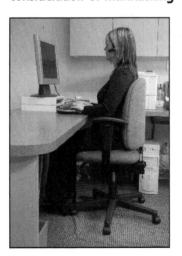

The seated posture that places the least stress on the spine is slightly reclined (about 10 degrees), with the hip angle opened to about 100 degrees.[4] While it is possible to drive a car or fly to space in this position, it is difficult to practice dentistry in this manner, due to the need to view the oral cavity. It is also inconvenient for most dental front office workers to utilize this position due to multitasking, which frequently requires workers to leave their work stations or view paperwork on their desks. Positioning and equipment selection for the dental front office should consider the many duties performed by these individuals: computer entry, answering phones, billing, scheduling appointments, filling out insurance claim forms, completing paperwork, and filing charts. (Fig. 1)

# Office Chairs

Although most dental front office executives are female, the majority of office chairs are designed for the average European man. Walk into any generic office store looking for office chairs, and you will find many large, cushy office chairs, with tall backs, no lumbar support, and reclining tilt features. These office "thrones" that reflect authority are a vestige of years gone past, when important political figures required large thrones with high backs to reflect status. Unfortunately, most ergonomic considerations (if there ever were any) went out the window with this chair style. This chair design poses two primary problems for most female front office personnel: deep seat pans and insufficient lumbar support.

You should be able to sit all the way back in your office chair and easily place three finger widths between the back of your knee and the seat. If you cannot, your seat pan may be too deep, causing you to perch on the edge of your seat. (Fig. 2) This will quickly fatigue low back muscles, and may lead to low-back pain. The average height woman will be most comfortable in about a 16-inch deep seat pan, which may be difficult to find at generic office stores.[1] You will find free reviews for various front office chairs at *www.posturedontics.com*, under "Product Reviews."

**Fig. 2: Large, executive-style chairs frequently have deep seat pans, causing shorter to average-height workers to perch on the edge of the chair**

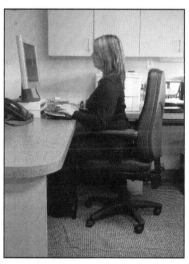

The chair should also have an adjustable lumbar support that tilts forward and adjusts up and down so the most convex portion nestles in the low back curve. Unlike their dental colleagues in the operatories, most front office workers are able to maintain contact with their lumbar supports for a majority of their working hours. This is probably why we see less low-back pain among

**Fig. 3: An adjustable lumbar support can be mounted to non-ergonomic chairs**

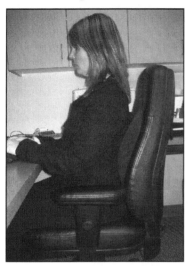

office workers than among dental professionals. Chairs without a lumbar support may be retrofitted with a small lumbar cushion to attain proper spinal alignment and support. (Fig. 3)

A backward (reclining) tilt feature on the seat pan can allow for maximum relaxation of the lumbar musculature and spinal discs during break periods[5] but will encourage poor spinal alignment and forward head posture if utilized during desk work. The seat pan should adjust slightly forward to allow the individual to sit with thighs sloping very slightly downward. This helps to facilitate the lumbar curve.[6] Chairs that have a non-tilting seat pan may be retrofitted with an ergonomic wedge-shaped cushion (Chapter 3), which may also help prevent or resolve sciatic pain in some individuals.

Armrests have also been shown to decrease neck and shoulder strain. It is important to make sure the design and height adjustment of the armrests do not cause them to hit the counter.

Chair selection criteria and adjustment are similar to those for dental operator stools. (Chapters 2 and 6) The front office chair should be adjusted before measuring or adjusting any other equipment, as described in Chapter 2, with the following additions.

After finishing chair adjustment, if you cannot rest your weight through your feet flat on the floor, use a footrest to support the feet.

# Keyboards and Keyboard Trays

After adjusting the chair, the keyboard height should be determined. Unfortunately, the height of the front office counter or desk is usually nonadjustable. Neck and shoulder pain, especially trapezius myalgia (Chapter 4) can result from keyboards placed on a counter that is too high.[1] On the other hand, keyboards that are too low will cause the individual's shoulders and head to slump forward, and wrists may be bent up.

Make sure your keyboard facilitates a relaxed posture of the arm with elbow at side and the forearm level or sloping slightly downward.[7] The angle of the keyboard should facilitate a straight, or neutral, wrist posture when viewed from the side. (Fig. 1)

If you notice your wrists are bent upward when your hands are on your keyboard on a fixed-height counter, try lowering the legs on the back of the keyboard to make it flat. If your forearms are angled upward, install an inclined keyboard tray under the countertop (Fig. 4) and angle it downward to facilitate a straight wrist posture. Inclined keyboard trays frequently solve both keyboard height problems and wrist angle problems.

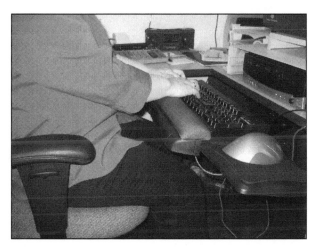

**Fig. 4: An inclined keyboard tray frequently resolves both height and wrist posture problems**

A wrist rest should be just that—a rest. Using the wrist rest to support the wrists while actively typing can compress the carpal tunnel and lead to pain syndromes.

Keyboard styles vary. Traditional keyboard designs encourage non-neutral wrist position, bending the wrist toward the little finger. This can lead to tendonitis. Ergonomic keyboards place the keys in a diagonal slope to facilitate neutral wrist position.

# Monitors

Due to an inherent need to see incoming patients, monitors are often placed to one side of the keyboard, causing the front office executive to work with the head turned to one side. Combine this with the "phone shoulder holder" habit (Fig. 5), and you have a recipe for a musculoskeletal disaster. In this case, intervention is not an option, it is a must. Make sure monitors are always placed directly behind the keyboard. If space is a consideration, it may be time to upgrade to a flat-screen monitor.

**Fig. 5: A recipe for musculoskeletal disaster: holding the phone between the shoulder and ear with the monitor off to one side**

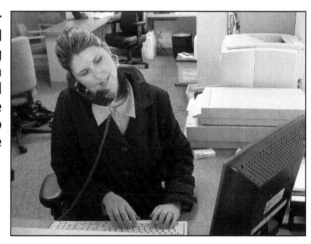

Working with the monitor too high or too low can result in neck pain. The top of the monitor *screen* should be at or slightly below eye level.[7] Have someone evaluate this from the side, while sitting in a chair. Most frequently, I find the monitor is positioned too low. Monitor risers may be placed under the monitor to raise the monitor to the proper working level.(Fig. 1) The monitor should be about 18 inches to 24 inches away from the worker's eyes.

Monitors should be placed so that the worker's line of sight is parallel to outside (natural) light coming through a window. Overhead lighting should be indirect and not cause glare on the screen. Direct lighting (a small desk light) may be helpful to illuminate paperwork and keyboard.[7]

## FRONT OFFICE PERSPECTIVES

Practice administrator and 29-year veteran, Deanna Alexander of Lansing, Mich., learned the importance of prevention the hard way. She states, "After working for 25 years with the phone cradled between my shoulder and ear, I developed pain in my arm and hand, with numbness into my fourth and fifth fingers. I consider phone headsets a must for every front office."

"Chronic pain lowers one's positive attitude," says Joan Oriard, an administrative coordinator in Airway Heights, Wash., for more than 20 years. "This could affect your interoffice relationships and work performance."

Ms. Alexander concurs. "Poor front office ergonomics has definitely negatively affected my productivity." She applauds those dentists (including her own), who value their front office team and invest in ergonomic changes.

Ms. Oriard has never experienced chronic work-related pain. When asked what her secret is, she credited, "A good ergonomic chair, proper desk height, daily walking and exercise."

# Work Space

A frequent problem in the dental front office is placing paperwork in front of the keyboard, which causes excessive reaching, slouching and forward head posture. Always place the keyboard close enough so the elbows are relaxed at the sides while typing. Copy and other paperwork may be placed to one side on a copy holder, at the monitor screen height.

# Wireless Phone Headsets

Perhaps the most dangerous of all front office risk factors is holding the phone between one shoulder and ear. (Fig. 5) Why do so many front office people do this? Simple—because people don't have three hands. The phone conversation typically involves the computer, which requires both hands. Invariably, this habit will eventually cause neck and shoulder pain on one side of the body. An easy and comfortable solution is the wireless phone headset. (Fig. 1) This can be worn over one ear, and calls may be answered from afar in the office through a remote phone lifter device.[1]

# Mouse Reaching

Ideally, your computer mouse should be placed at the same level as the keyboard to eliminate excessive reaching, or, worse, repeatedly reaching up and out to the mouse. This can lead to pain in the "mousing" shoulder. Frequently these individuals will find the shoulder blade on the mousing shoulder has shifted upward when compared with the opposite side.

A simple solution to this is a "mouse bridge," which can attach to many keyboard platforms and either slides underneath the platform or attaches on the side. (Fig. 6)

**Fig. 6: A common mistake is placing the mouse at a different level than the keyboard. This can be resolved with a mouse bridge**

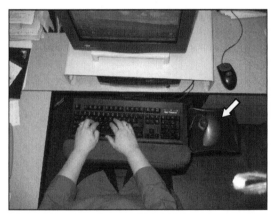

# Dualing Mice

Repeatedly using the same mouse can result in fatigue and pain in the intrinsic hand muscles and tendons. Try alternating between a thumb-trackball mouse and a regular mouse. (Fig. 7) This will avoid overworking one area of the hand and wrist. Plug one mouse into your US/2 port, and the other into a USB port, so you can easily switch between the two during the work day.

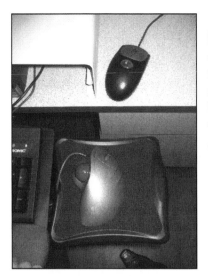

**Fig. 7: Alternating between a regular mouse and a thumb track-ball mouse may help prevent certain types of tendonitis in the hand by moving the workload to different areas of the hand**

# Stretching

To diminish the cumulative negative impact of static posturing in the front office, it is important to incorporate regularly scheduled microbreaks throughout the day. (Chapter 2) These have been shown to reduce computer operator discomfort, while having no detrimental impact on productivity.[8] Consider stretching while you are "on hold" on the phone, waiting for the computer, between patients or at stop lights while driving home.

Just as in dental ergonomics, an effective front office ergonomics program involves addressing numerous areas. The impact of improving your front office can have numerous ramifications: improved attitude, productivity and interoffice relationships. Consider that your front office personnel are a mirror reflection of your practice. The tact, professionalism and patience required of these individuals are easily compromised by discomfort or pain. This attitude, in turn, is undoubtedly perceived by your patients.

Dentists will quickly recognize the benefits reaped from "ergonomizing" their front offices for a happy, more profitable and comfortable front office team.

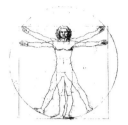

# Putting it
# into Practice

Even if you're on the right track,
you'll get run over if you just sit there.

WILL ROGERS

By now, you may have surmised a central tenet of a prevention program. To be effective in the long-term, prevention strategies must become a lifestyle habit. This may involve a paradigm shift in your dental practice and methods of operating. If prevention strategies are implemented only during times of physical duress, the process of accumulated microtrauma increases your risk of sustaining permanent structural damage.

The accrual of knowledge is of little value without a system to practice and implement it, which is why you had clinics in dental school. Likewise, it can be overwhelming to absorb and attempt to implement the large volume of information in this book. Following is a system to help you effectively implement the strategies in this book to optimize your results.

## Start small

Select only two strategies to begin with. If you are experiencing discomfort, these strategies should probably be from the chapter that corresponds to your area of pain. If you are coming from a preventive standpoint, start with Chapter 2, and be sure your posture and position are well-supported in the operatory. Allow yourself to become comfortable with the new strategies until they have become habit (usually about 1 month). Then you may introduce 1 or 2 new strategies, as needed.

## Cut costs

Before purchasing expensive ergonomic equipment, explore less-expensive alternate methods to resolve an ergonomic problem. Oftentimes, ergonomic solutions don't cost a dime! Think "outside the box" to achieve space in which to operate, retrieve instruments and move freely around the patient. Adjust operator stools, rotate patient chairs, reposition the assistant and, yes...even move the patient chair as much as 10 inches to 12 inches to achieve your desired ergonomic goal. *(Always check with the manufacturer before moving the patient chair, and always recruit several strong bodies to team up in the effort!)*

## Start stretching

After you have tried the Chairside Stretches in Chapter 2, determine which ones, and in which direction you were tightest. Select only two stretches to begin with, and decide *when* you will implement them during the day. Associating the stretch with a particular procedure (i.e., while assistant is light curing, waiting for anesthesia, during a failed appointment) will make it easier to remember during the day. Add 1 or 2 more stretches after these have become habit.

## *Post it*

Place your stretching wall charts or other visual cue in your opera-tory in clear view so you remember to implement the strategy throughout the workday.

## *Take it slow*

When beginning any new strategy, especially those with a significant impact on the musculoskeletal system, it is important to begin with the minimum to avoid overuse and subsequent discomfort. For loupes, this means perhaps only 2 hours of wear per day for 3 to 4 days. For stretching, this means gently working into the beginning of the stretch. For saddle stools, this may mean only 2 to 3 hours of daily use during the first week.

## *Consider consulting*

If your ergonomic challenges are too overwhelming, or you wish for an expert's opinion, consider hiring a dental ergonomic consult-ant. As with all professions, there will be a range of capabilities. Most important, look for someone who specializes in dentistry, then look for accreditation with dental associations (ADA, AGD), and also research-based publications in dental journals.

## *Knowledge is power!*

There is much more education to be attained than could possibly be included in this book. There are many expert clinicians and doctors who lecture on health. Take advantage of these educational opportunities whenever possible. To safeguard your own health, insist on research-based information in seminars, articles and other information products.

## *Take time*

Remember that pain and postural problems usually develop over years and years. Resolution of these issues is typically not instantaneous, but may take 2 or 3 weeks of consistent implementation until you see results. Most importantly, be patient—change is rarely comfortable.

As I write this, my ultimate business goal is beginning to materialize: several dental schools in the United States are now implementing mandatory ergonomic programs into their dental school curriculum and testing on ergonomic concepts. Numerous dental hygiene schools have already done so. This is a sign of changing times, astute forethought and wise decision-making in dental and hygiene school administration. With rising awareness of the prevalence of this problem, and strategic, early interventions, my hope is that there will be far fewer early retirees and countless operators who will practice dentistry in comfort for as long as they desire.

You have invested a great amount of time and money into your professional career. Practicing early prevention strategies is one of the best insurance policies you can implement to ensure your own musculoskeletal health and career longevity. After all, what good is your lucrative dental practice if your body retires before you do?

# Ergonomic Resources
# for Dental Professionals

This appendix provides valuable resources to aid team members in implementing ergonomic changes in their offices and treating chronic pain. You will find resources for dental ergonomic products, manufacturers, articles, books, consultants, education, healthcare professionals and other health products. The product listing is not intended to be a complete listing of all dental products available, but those that the author has found to be beneficial from an ergonomic perspective in dental ergonomic consultations and also in clinical trials. Due to anthropometric and health variances between individuals, the listed products are not official recommendations, and dental professionals are urged to carefully research any product to see if it is a proper fit for themselves and their office.

Please note that addresses are current just before going to press; however, website addresses and URLs are constantly updated and changing. If you find a URL is not valid, do an online search by name for the product/service.

## Books/Articles

*All the Right Moves: The definitive guide for integrating dental team ergonomics, treatment room technology, auxiliary utilization and office design,* by Risa Pollack-Simon

*Ergonomic benefits of surgical telescope systems: selection guidelines* by B.J. Chang. CDA Journal, February 2002

*Ergonomic requirements for dental equipment: Guidelines and recommendations for designing, constructing and selecting dental equipment,* by Hokwerda, Wouters and de Ruijter. Available at *www.optergo.com*

*Ergonomics and the Dental Care Worker,* by Denise C. Murphy

*Four-Handed Dentistry: A handbook of clinical application and ergonomic Concepts,* by Betty Ladley Finkbeiner (includes operator positioning chart for specific tooth surfaces/quadrants of the mouth)

*It's Not Carpal Tunnel Syndrome!,* by Suparna Damany and Jack Bellis

*Low Back Disorders: Evidence-based prevention and rehabilitation,* by Stuart McGill

*Painfree: A revolutionary method for stopping chronic pain,* by Pete Egoscue

*Sports Injury Prevention & Rehabilitation,* by Shamus & Shamus

*The Mindbody Prescription: Healing the body, healing the pain,* by John Sarno

*The Relaxation & Stress Reduction Workbook,* by Davis/Eschelman/McKay

*The Trigger Point Therapy Workbook: Your self-treatment guide for pain relief,* by Clair Davies

*Treat Your Own Neck,* by Robin McKenzie

*Understand your Backache: A guide to prevention, treatment and relief,* by Rene Cailliet

# CDs

*The Ultimate Back: Assessment and therapeutic exercise,* by Stuart McGill

*Journey into Deep Relaxation,* by Doreen Blumenfeld
*Delta Sleep System,* by Jeffrey Thompson

# Dental Ergonomic Consulting

David Ahearn, DDS: Design Ergonomics: *www.design-ergonomics.com* (office design)

Tim Caruso, PT, MBA: *carusopt@ameritech.net*

Ergolinks, *www.ergolinks.biz*

Mary Govoni, CDA, RDH: *www.marygovoni.com.*

Bethany Valachi, PT, MS: Posturedontics LLC: *www.posturedontics.com*

# Dental Hygienist Seminars/CDs

### PERIODONTAL INSTRUMENTATION SEMINARS

Anna Pattison, Jill Rethman, et al.: www.*dimensionsofdentalhygiene.com*

Esther Wilkins/Anna Pattison: *www.internationaldentalseminars.com*

### ULTRASONIC SEMINARS

Anne Guignon, RDH, MPH: *www.ergosonics.com*

### INSTRUMENT SHARPENING TECHNIQUE CD

Dianne Glasscoe, RDH: *www.professionaldentalmgmt.com*

# Dental Product Reviews

Dr. Christianson's CRA Newsletter: *www.cranews.com*

DentalCompare: *www.DentalCompare.com*

Posturedontics, LLC: *www.posturedontics.com*
(ergonomic products only)

Reality Publishing Company: *www.realityesthetics.com*

# Dental Ergonomic Products: Operatory

### ARMRESTS

ErgoRest articulating arm support. Multiple vendors online

## ASSISTANT STOOLS

*(Recommend torso support bar-only or backrest-only designs)*

*Adec:* 1600 series: *www.a-dec.com*

*Brewer:* 3145R/L: *www.brewer-design.com*

*DentalEZ:* Premium series: *www.dentalez.com*

*Dentech:* Ergotilt: *www.dentechcorp.com*

*Marus:* DC5010 and 5110 only: *www.marus.com*

*Midmark:* Stool w/o backrest: *www.midmark.com*

*Pelton & Crane:* 2004 model: *www.pelton.net*

## DELIVERY SYSTEMS (REAR, SIDE AND OVER-THE-PATIENT)

Available through most dental suppliers

## DELIVERY SYSTEM: OVER-THE-HEAD

Design Ergonomics: *www.ergonomic-products.com*

## ERGONOMIC SEAT CUSHIONS

*Fit-Sit* ergonomic seat cushion: *www.posturedontics.com*

## GLOVES—FITTED

*Smart Practice:* QualiTouch Fitted L/R: *www.smartpractice.com*

## LIGHTING SYSTEMS

Loupe-mounted headlamps: Most loupe manufacturers

Isolite Dryfield Illuminator: *www.isolitesystems.com*

Mirroscope: *www.miras-imaging.com*

## MAGNIFICATION—TELESCOPES/LOUPES

Heine: *www.heine.com*

Orascoptic: *www.orascoptic.com*

SurgiTel Systems: *www.surgitel.com*

Perioptix: *www.perioptix.com*

Seiler: *www.seilerinst.com*

## MAGNIFICATION—MICROSCOPES
Global: *www.globalsurgical.com*
Seiler: *www.seilerinst.com*
Zeiss: *www.zeiss.com*

## MAGNIFICATION—PROCEDURE SCOPES
MagnaVu: *www.magnifiedvideodentistry.com*

## MISCELLANEOUS ERGONOMIC EQUIPMENT
The Wand/CompuDent anesthetic delivery:
*www.milestonescientific.com*
Automix impression material device: *www.products3.3m.com*
Mirror suction: *www.panadent.com*

## OPERATOR STOOLS
*Brewer Design:* Alleviate & EG series: *www.brewer-design.com*
*CoreWerks:* CoreBalance Stool: *www.propriotek.com*
*Crown Seating:* 30 series hygienist: *www.crownseating.com*
*Crown Seating:* 70/80 series dentist: *www.crownseating.com*
*DentalEZ:* Generation series: *www.dentalez.com*
*Dentech Corp:* Advance: *www.dentechcorp.com*
*Link Dental Corp:* Doctor series: *www.linkdental.com*
*Orascoptic:* Bodyguard Chair: *www.orascoptic.com*
*Pelton & Crane:* Model 2003: *www.pelton.net*
*PosturePerfect:* Evolution Ball Chair: *www.evolutionchair.com*
*RGP:* Swedish chair (highly contoured seat): *www.rgpdental.com*
*Royal Dental:* All models except RO2: *www.royaldentalgroup.com*
*Saddle stool:* Bambach: *www.hagerworldwide.com*
*Saddle stool:* Salli: *www.salli.com*
*Saddle stool:* Scandex: *www.scandex.us*

**PATIENT CHAIRS**

*DentalEZ:* JV Generation Chair: *www.dentalez.com*

*Dentech Corp:* Eco19 Chair: *www.dentechcorp.com*

*Pelton & Crane:* Spirit 3004 Chair: *www.pelton.net*

*Royal Dental:* Domain & Signet Chairs: *www.royaldentalgroup.com*

**PATIENT POSITIONING AIDS**

Crescent Dental Products: *www.crescentproducts.com* (memory foam headrest, backrest, knee support, pedo-booster and geriatric headrest)

**SCRUBS**

Scrub Med: *www.scrubmed.com*

**TECHNOLOGY**

Dental Technology Consultants: *www.thedigitaldentist.com*

Dental Systems Integrators Inc.: *www.dentalsystemsintegrators.com*

**ULTRASONIC SCALERS/HAND INSTRUMENTS**

Ultrasonic inserts–swivel: *www.hu-friedy.com*

Ultrasonic inserts–large diameter: *www.premusa.com*

Hand Instruments: www.hu-friedy.com, *www.am-eagle.com*

Wide grip instruments: *www.hu-friedy.com*

# Ergonomic Products: Front Office

**COMPUTER STATION PRODUCTS**

(available at most office stores or online)

Gel-filled wrist rests for keyboard, mousepads

Vu Ryser monitor stand (elevates monitor)

Copy holder – holds written material

Phone headsets – (*not* a shoulder cradle!)

Ergonomic pen/pencil grips – many types

Footrest (for stations being used by persons of different heights)

Under desk mouse platform

Under counter keyboard tray system

Thumb-operated trackball mouse

## LUMBAR SUPPORTS

*Chair lumbar Support:* McKenzie SuperRoll: *www.optp.com*

Other lumbar supports (chair and car seats): *www.backdesigns.com*
*www.healthyback.com*

## FRONT OFFICE CHAIRS

Global Granada multifunction office chair:
*www.officechairsunlimited.com*

Bodybilt custom chairs: *www.ergo4me.com*

Zody office chair: *www.haworth.com*

Joakim swivel chair: *www.ikea.com*

Leap chair: *www.humanscale.com*

Hag office chairs: *www.sitincomfort.com*

Raynor Patriot multifunction task chair: Office Depot

## ERGONOMIC FLOOR MATS (LAB)

Ergomat: *www.ergomat.com*

Ergonomic anti-fatigue mats: *www.ergosource.com*

# Injury Prevention Products

Backnobber (trigger point self-treatment tool):
*www.posturedontics.com*

*Trigger Point Therapy Workbook* by Davies:
*www.posturedontics.com*

## HOT/COLD PACKS

Apollo Paks (Velcro, reusable): *www.thesaundersgroup.com*

Icy Hot Heat Therapy (disposable): *www.icyhot.com*

## POSTURAL

Posture S'Port (body support undergarment): *www.posturedontics.com*

## WRIST HEALTH

WrisTimer (carpal tunnel prevention): *www.posturedontics.com*

## EXERCISE FOR DENTAL PROFESSIONALS

Home Exercise DVD Package for dental professionals: *www.posturedontics.com*

Chairside Stretching & Trigger Point DVD Package: *www.posturedontics.com*

Swiss Exercise Balls: *www.posturedontics.com*

Rubber Exercise Tubing: *www.posturedontics.com*

## SLEEP

Select Comfort *Sleep Number* air bed: *www.selectcomfort.com*

Tempurpedic mattresses: *www.tempurpedic.com*

Tempurpedic NeckPillow: *www.tempurpedic.com*

# Glossary

**Abduction.** To move away from the midline of the body.

**Aerobic.** Using oxygen to enhance respiratory and circulatory efficiency.

**Anthropometric.** Pertaining to the measurement of the size and proportions of the human body.

**Autogenics.** Self-induced relaxation technique which influences the autonomic nervous system.

**Biomechanics.** The study of the forces exerted by muscles and gravity on the skeletal structure.

**Body mechanics.** The use of kinesiological principles to facilitate proper body movement, and to prevent and correct postural and endurance problems.

**Buccal.** Pertaining to the cheek side of the mouth.

**Carpal tunnel syndrome.** Chronic pain, numbness, or tingling in the hand, caused by compression of the median nerve at the wrist. Can be caused by occupational risk factors or medical conditions.

**Carrier lens.** The larger lens on dental telescopes. In TTL loupes, the scope is mounted directly into the carrier lens.

**Cervical radiculopathy.** Irritation or compression of a nerve root in the neck as it leaves the spinal canal. Pain is referred distally into the shoulder, arm and hand.

**Cubital tunnel syndrome.** The most common form of ulnar nerve entrapment at the elbow, referring pain, numbness or tingling into the ring and small fingers.

**Cumulative trauma disorder (CTD).** Work-related pain or injury to the musculoskeletal system resulting from microtrauma which accumulates at a rate faster than the body can repair it (a.k.a. MSD (musculoskeletal disorder), RSI (repetitive strain injury), RMI (repetitive motion injury), RTI (repetitive trauma injury).

**Declination angle.** In dental loupes, the steepness at which the scope is angled downward on the loupes.

**deQuervain's syndrome.** Inflammation of the sheath or tunnel that surrounds the two tendons that control movement of the thumb. Stabbing pain is felt on the thumb side of the wrist.

**Delivery system.** Unit that holds dental handpieces and instruments in close proximity for easy retrieval.

**Ergonomics.** The application of human physiology to the design of objects, systems and environment to maximize worker productivity and reduce injuries.

**Herniated disc.** The extrusion of the inner nucleus through the wall of a degenerated spinal disc. This often causes painful compression on spinal nerves.

**Hypermobility** (also double-jointedness or hyperlaxity). Joint movement that stretches farther than is normal.

**Hypomobility.** Limited movement, or stiffness in joints.

**Ischemia.** A decrease in the blood supply to a body part caused by constriction or obstruction of the blood vessels.

**Kinesiology.** The scientific study of human body movment; how muscles act and coordinate to move the body.

**Kyphosis.** Natural convex curve in the thoracic spine. Severe kyphosis can be congenital or a result of poor posture.

**Labial.** Pertaining to the lip side of the mouth.

**Lateral epicondylitis.** Inflammation of the tendon at the outside of the elbow resulting from overuse of forearm muscles.

**Lordosis.** Natural concave curve in the cervical and lumbar spine. Severe lordosis (hyperlordosis) involves an abnormal forward curvature of the lumbar spine, resulting in a swaybacked posture.

**Loupes (telescopes).** Magnification glasses worn by dental professionals and surgeons while operating.

**Mobile cart.** A cart on wheels that houses dental supplies, which may include instrumentation, materials and handpieces. Most often used by assistants.

**Mover muscles.** Muscles that are designed for power and are located farther from the center of the body.

**Myalgia.** Muscle pain.

**Microtrauma.** Physiological microscopic damage that occurs in the musculoskeletal system due to numerous ergonomic risk factors.

**Muscle adaptation.** Over time, the adaptive shortening and lengthening of muscles to accommodate prolonged, unbalanced body postures.

**Muscle substitution.** Secondary muscles performing a job for which they are not designed, due to compromised function of the primary muscle group.

**Muscle imbalance.** Response to unbalanced posture. Groups of muscles become long and weak, while the opposing muscle groups become short and strong, holding the body in non-neutral posture.

**Myofascial.** Fascia separating and surrounding muscle tissue.

**Occlusal.** Biting or chewing surfaces of the teeth.

**Operatory.** Patient treatment rooms in the dental office.

**Prolonged static posture (PSP).** A primary risk factor contributing to microtrauma in dentistry.

**Pronator teres syndrome.** Compression of the median nerve in the proximal forearm, often due to trigger points. Can mimic carpal tunnel syndrome.

**Proprioception.** The unconscious sense of the position, location, orientation and movement of the body and its parts.

**Radial tunnel syndrome.** Compression of a branch of the radial nerve in the forearm, referring pain to the forearm and lateral side of the elbow.

**Rotator cuff impingement.** Painful tendonitis of the supraspinatus tendon in the shoulder due to repetitive lifting, overhead reaching or abduction.

**Spondylosis.** A degenerative disease of the spine, leading to fusion and immobilization of the vertebral bones.

**Stabilizer muscles.** Muscles designed for endurance and stability, located closer to the spine of the body.

**Target heart rate.** Calculation for determining safe aerobic exercise levels.

**Tendonitis.** Inflammation of a tendon.

**Tension neck syndrome.** Pain and tenderness in the cervical musculature, usually due to poor ergonomic conditions.

**Thoracic outlet syndrome.** A neurovascular disease causing compression of the nerves and artery that supply the arm and hand. Symptoms include numbness, weakness, pain, discoloration or coldness.

**Torso support bar.** Movable, C-shaped bar on the assistant stool.

**Trapezius myalgia.** Pain and tenderness in the upper trapezius muscle, often due to prolonged shoulder elevation or emotional stress.

**Trigger point.** Painful, palpable cluster of muscle fibers in a sustained contraction, due to postural asymmetry, accidents, poor ergonomic conditions, muscle ischemia and other risk factors.

# References

## Chapter One

1. Akesson I, Johnsson B, Rylander L, Moritz U, Skerfving S. Musculoskeletal disorders among female dental personnel – clinical examination and a 5-year follow-up study of symptoms. *Int Arch Occup Environ Health* 1999;72:395-403.

2. Akesson I, Schutz A, Horstmann V, Skerfving S, Moritz U. Musculoskeletal symptoms among dental personnel; – lack of association with mercury and selenium status, overweight and smoking. *Swed Dental J* 2000;24:23-28.

3. Alexopoulos EC, Stathi I, Charizani F. Prevalence of musculoskeletal disorders in dentists. *BMC Musculoskelet Disord* 2004;5:16.

4. Auguston TE, Morken T. Musculoskeletal problems among dental health personnel. A survey of the public dental health services in Hordaland. *Tdsskr Nor Laegeforen*. 1996;116(23):2776-80.

5. Chowanadisai S, Kukiattrakoon B, Yapong B, Kedjarune U. Occupational health problems of dentists in southern Thailand. *Int Dent J* 2000;50:36-40.

6. Fish DR, Morris-Allen DM. Musculoskeletal disorders in dentists. *NY State Dent J* 1998;64(4):44-48.

7. Finsen L, Christensen H, Bakke M. Musculoskeletal disorders among dentists and variation in dental work. *Applied Ergonomics* 1997;29(2):119-125.

8. Lalumandier J, McPhee S, Parrott C, Vendemia M. Musculoskeletal pain: Prevalence, prevention, and differences among dental office personnel. *General Dentistry* 2001;49:160-6.

9. Lalumandier J, McPhee S. Prevalence and risk factors of hand problems and carpal tunnel syndrome among dental hygienists. *J Dent Hyg* 2001; 75:130-133.

10. Lehto TU, Helenius HY, Alaranta HT. Musculoskeletal symptoms of dentists assessed by a multidisciplinary approach. *Community Dent Oral Epidemiol* 1991;19:38-44.

11. Marshall ED, Duncombe LM, Robinson RQ, Kilbreath, SL. Musculoskeletal symptoms in New South Wales dentists. *Aust Dent J* 1997;42(4):240-6.

12. Osborn JB, Newell KJ, Rudney JD, Stoltenberg JL. Musculoskeletal pain among Minnesota dental hygienists. *J Dent Hyg* 1990;64(3):132-8.

13. Ratzon NZ, Yaros T, Mizlik A, Kanner T. Musculoskeletal symptoms among dentists in relation to work posture. *Work* 2000;15:153-8.

14. Rucker LM, Sunell S. Ergonomic Risk Factors Associated with Clinical Dentistry. *CDA J* 2002;30(2):139-48.

15. Rundcrantz B, Johnsson B, Moritz U. Cervical pain and discomfort among dentists. Epidemiological, clinical and therapeutic aspects. *Swed Dent J* 1990;14:71-80.

16. Rundcrantz B, Johnsson B, Moritz U. Occupational cervico-brachial disorders among dentists: Analysis of ergonomics and locomotor functions. *Swed Dent J* 1991;15:105-15.

17. Shenkar O, Mann J, Shevach A, Ever-Hadani P, Weiss P. Prevalence and risk factors of upper extremity cumulative trauma disorder in dental hygienists. *Work* 1998;11:263-75.

18. Shugars DA, Miller D, Williams D, Fishburne C, Strickland D. Musculoskeletal pain among general dentists. *Gen Dent* 1987;35:272-6.

19. Biller FE. Occupational hazards in dental practice. *Oral Hygiene* 1946; 36:1994.

20. Rising DW, Bennett BC, Hursh K, Plesh O. Reports of body pain in a dental student population. *JADA* 2005;136:81-86.

21. Morse T, Bruneau H, Michalak-Turcotte C, Sanders M, Warren N, Dussetschleger J, Diva U, Croteau M, Cherniack M. Musculoskeletal disorders of the neck and shoulder in dental hygienists and dental hygiene students. *J Dent Hyg* 2007;81(1):10.

22. Valachi B, Valachi K. Mechanisms contributing to musculoskeletal disorders in dentistry. *J Am Dent Assoc* 2003;134(10):1344-50.

23. 2005 Survey of Dental Practice: Income from the private practice of dentistry. Chicago, Ill.:*ADA Survey Center* 2007.

24. Burke FJ, Main JR, Freeman R. The practice of dentistry: an assessment of reasons for premature retirement. *Br Dent J* 1997;182(7):250-4.

25. Back and cervical disabilities sideline dentists most often. Chicago, Ill.: *ADA News*; Dec 2005;8.

26. Carter T. What are you worth? *Modern Hygienist* 2007;4:2-4.

27. Kane M. Kane Insurance Services Inc. [Personal interview]. January 18, 2007.

28. Miller DL. An investigation into attrition of dental hygienists from the work force. *J Dent Hyg* 1991;65(1):25-31.

29. Pope M. Muybridge Lecture, International Society of Biomechanics XIVth Congress. Paris, France. July 1993.

30. Pope MH, Goh KL, Magnusson ML. Spine Ergonomics. *Annu Rev Biomed Eng* 2002;4:49-68.

31. Kihara T. Dental care works and work-related complaints of dentists. *Kurume Medical Journal* 1995;42:251-257.

32. Saunders H, Saunders R. *Evaluations, Treatment and Prevention of Musculoskeletal Disorders,* Vol 1. Minnesota: Educational Opportunities, A Saunders Group Company 1995;47,100-101.

33. Chaitow L, Delany JW. *Clinical application of neuromuscular techniques. Vol 1: the upper body.* Philadelphia:Elsevier Science 2003:55-57.

34. Kroemer K, Grandjean E. *Fitting the task to the human, 5$^{th}$ ed.* Philadelphia:Taylor & Francis 1997:8.

35. Kumar C. *Biomechanics in Ergonomics*. Philadelphia: Taylor & Francis 1999;12.

36. Cailliet R. *Soft Tissue Pain and Disability. 3ʳᵈ ed*. Philadelphia: F.A. Davis Company 1996;71-72.

37. Karwowski W, Marras W. *The Occupational Ergonomics Handbook*. Florida: CRC Press LLC 1999;255.

38. Travell JG, Simons DG, Simons LS. Myofascial Pain and Dysfunction: *The Trigger Point Manual, Vol. 1*. Baltimore, Maryland: Lippincott Williams & Wilkins 1999;4,12,19,35,329-396.

39. Guay AH. The American Dental Association and dental ergonomics: Research, observations and activities. In: Murphy, DC (Ed), *Ergonomics and the dental care worker*. Washington: American Public Health Association 1998.

40. Melis M, About-Atme YS, Cottogno L, Pittau R. Upper body musculoskeletal symptoms in Sardinian dental students. *J Can Dent Assoc* 2004 May;70(5):306-310.

41. Tezel A, Kavrut F, Tezel A, Kara C, Demir T, Kavrut R. Musculoskeletal disorders in left- and right-handed Turkish dental students. *Int J Neurosci*. 2005;115(2):255-66.

42. Beach JC, DeBiase CB. Assessment of ergonomic education in dental hygiene curricula. *J Dent Educ* 1998;62(6):421-5.

43. Thornton LJ, Stuart-Buttle C, Wyszynski TC, Wilson ER. Physical and psychosocial stress exposures in US dental schools: the need for expanded ergonomics training. *Applied Ergonomics* 2004;35:153-7.

44. Connelly E, Propst S. 2005 investment in US health research. *Research!America*: Available at *www.researchamerica.org/advocacy/ healthresearchinvestment.html*

45. Pillastrini P, Mugnai R, Farneti C, Bertozzi L, Bonfiglioli R, et al. Evaluation of two preventive interventions for reducing musculoskeleletal complaints in operators of video display terminals. *Physical Therapy* 2007;87(5):536-544.

46. Droeze EH, Jonsson H. Evaluation of ergonomic interventions to reduce musculoskeletal disorders of dentists in the Netherlands. *Work* 2005;25(3):221-20.

47. Goodman G, Landis J, George C, McGuire S, Shorter C, Sieminski M, Wilson T. Effectiveness of computer ergonomics interventions for an engineering company: a program evaluation. *Work* 2005;24(1):53-62.

48. Nelson A, Matz M, Chen F, Siddharthan K, Lloyd J, Fragala G. Development and evaluation of a multifaceted ergonomics program to prevent injuries associated with patient handling tasks. *Int J Nurs Stud* 2006;43(6):717-33.

49. Fujishiro K, Weaver JL, Heaney CA, Hamrick CA, Marras WS. The effect of ergonomic interventions in healthcare facilities on musculoskeletal disorders. *Am J Ind Med* 2005;48(5):338-47.

50. McSweeney KP, Craig BN, Congleton JJ, Miller D. Ergonomic program effectiveness: ergonomic and medical intervention. *Int J Occup Saf Ergon* 2002;8(4):433-49.

51. Rivilis I, Cole DC, Frazer MB, Kerr MS, Wells RP, Ibrahim S. Evaluation of a participatory ergonomic intervention aimed at improving musculoskeletal health. *Am J Ind Med* 2006;49(10):801-10.

52. J W Collins, L Wolf, J Bell and B Evanoff. An evaluation of a "best practices" musculoskeletal injury prevention program in nursing homes. *Inj Prev* 2004;10:206-211

# Chapter Two

1. Saunders H, Saunders R. *Evaluation, Treatment and Prevention of Musculoskeletal Disorders, Vol 1*. Minnesota:Educational Opportunities, A Saunders Group Company 1995:7,46,147.

2. Chaitow L, Delany JW. *Clinical Application of Neuromuscular Techniques. Vol 1: the upper body*. Philadelphia: Elsevier Science 2003:29-41,52-53,57-58.

3. Rising DW, Bennett BC, Hursh K, Plesh O. Reports of body pain in a dental student population. *JADA* 2005;136:81-86.

4. Lee HY, Wang JD, Yao G, Wang SF. Association between cervicocephalic kinesthetic sensibility and frequency of subclinical neck pain. *Man Ther* 2007;1.

5. Revel M, Andre-Deshays C, Minguet M. Cervicocephalic kinesthetic sensibility in patients with cervical pain. *Arch Phys Med Rehabil* 1991;72(5):288-91.

6. Cailliet R. *Neck and Arm Pain. 3rd ed*. Philadelphia: F.A. Davis 1991:7, 43-50.

7. Ritter A, Sensat M, Harn, S. Thoracic Outlet Syndrome: A review of the literature. *Journal of Dental Hygiene* 1999;73:205-207.

8. Ferguson LW, Gerwin R. Clinical Mastery in the Treatment of Myofascial Pain. Baltimore: Lippincott Williams & Wilkins 2005:113-114.

9. Norkin C, Levangie P. The Vertebral Column. In: *Joint Structure and Function. A Comprehensive Analysis. 4th ed*. Philadelphia: F.A. Davis Company 2005.

10. Bogduk N. The inter-body joint and intervertebral discs. In: *Clinical anatomy of the lumbar spine and sacrum. 4th ed*. Philadelphia: Churchill Livingstone 2005.

11. Karwowski W, Marras W. *The Occupational Ergonomics Handbook*. Florida: CRC Press LLC 1999:175,184,1764-1784.

12. Chaffin D, Andersson G, Martin B. *Occupational Biomechanics. 3rd ed*. New York: John Wiley & Sons Inc 1999:355-391.

13. Chang B. Ergonomic Benefits of Surgical Telescope Systems: Selection Guidelines. *CDA Journal* 2002; 30(2):161-169.

14. Bridger RS, Wilkinson D, van Houweninge T. Hip joint mobility and spinal angles in standing and in different sitting postures. *Hum factors* 1989;31(2):229-41.

15. Bendix T, Biering-Sorensen F. Posture of the trunk when sitting on forward inclining seats. *Scand J Rehabil Med* 1983;15(4):197-203.

16. Rundcrantz B, Johnsson B, Moritz U. Cervical pain and discomfort among dentists. Epidemiological, clinical and therapeutic aspects. *Swed Dent J* 1990;14:71-80.

17. Finkbeiner BL. *Four-Handed Dentistry: A handbook of clinical application and ergonomic concepts.* New Jersey: Prentice Hall 2001.

18. Rundcrantz B, Johnsson B, Moritz U. Occupational cervico-brachial disorders among dentists: Analysis of ergonomics and locomotor functions. *Swed Dent J* 1991;15:105-15.

19. Steven W. White. Former president, Dentech Corporation. Personal interview, June 25, 2003.

20. Murphy D. *Ergonomics and the Dental Care Worker.* Washington, D.C.: American Public Health Association 1998:246-249,310-11.

21. Proteau R. Prevention of work-related musculoskeletal disorders in dental clinics. Montreal, Quebec: Association pour la sante et la securite; 2003. Available at: http://www.asstsas.qc.ca/english/publication.asp. Accessed July 31, 2007.

22. Valachi B, Valachi K. Mechanisms contributing to musculoskeletal disorders in dentistry. *Journal of the American Dental Association* 2003; Oct:134;1344-1350.

23. Lalumandier J, McPhee S, Parrott C, Vendemia M. Musculoskeletal pain: prevalence, prevention, and differences among dental office personnel. *Gen Dent* 2001;49:150-6.

24. Fish DR, Morris-Allen DM. Musculoskeletal disorders in dentists. *NY State Dent J* 1998;64(4):44-48.

25. Marshall ED, Duncombe LM, Robinson RQ, Kilbreath, SL. Musculoskeletal symptoms in New South Wales dentists. *Aust Dent J* 1997;42(4):240-6.

26. Finsen L, Christensen H, Bakke M. Musculoskeletal disorders among dentists and variation in dental work. *Applied Ergonomics* 1997;29(2):119-125.

27. Bandy WD, Irion JM, Briggler, M. The effect of static stretch and dynamic range of motion training on the flexibility of the hamstring muscles. *J Orthop Sports Phys Ther* 1998;27(4):295-300.

28. Roberts JM, Wilson K. Effect of stretching duration on active and passive range of motion in the lower extremity. *Br J Sports Med* 1999;33(4):259-63.

29. Cailliet R. *Soft Tissue Pain and Disability. 3rd ed.* Philadelphia: F.A. Davis Company 1996:71.

30. Kroemer K, Grandjean E. *Fitting the task to the human, 5th ed.* Philadelphia: Taylor & Francis 1997:8-10.

31. Travell JG, Simons DG, Simons LS. *Myofascial Pain and Dysfunction: The Trigger Point Manual, Vol. 1.* Baltimore, Maryland: Lippincott Williams & Wilkins 1999:135-8, 186.

32. McLean L, Tingley M, Scott R, Rickards J. Computer terminal work and the benefit of microbreaks. *Applied Ergonomics* 2001;32:225-237.

33. Kokkonen J, Nelson AG, Eldredge C, Winchester JB. Chronic static stretching improves exercise performance. *Med Sci Sports Exerc* 2007; 30(10):1825-31.

34. Rundcrantz B, Johnsson B, Moritz U. Occupational cervico-brachial disorders among dentists: Analysis of ergonomics and locomotor functions. *Swed Dent J* 1991;15:105-15.

35. Kihara T. Dental care works and work-related complaints of dentists. *Kurume Medical Journal* 1995;42:251-257.

# Chapter Three

1. Research on low back pain and common spinal disorders. *NIH Guide* 1997: 26(16). Available from: http://grants.nih.gov/grants/guide/pa-files/ PA-97-058.html (accessed August 2, 2007).

2. Karwowski W, Marras W. *The Occupational Ergonomics Handbook*. Florida: CRC Press LLC 1999;184,914,1765-66.

3. Rucker LM, Sunell S. Ergonomic Risk Factors Associated with Clinical Dentistry. *CDA J* 2002;30(2):139-48.

4. Finsen L, Christensen H, Bakke M. Musculoskeletal disorders among dentists and variation in dental work. *Applied Ergonomics* 1997;29(2):119-125.

5. Osborn JB, Newell KJ, Rudney JD, Stoltenberg JL. Musculoskeletal pain among Minnesota dental hygienists. *J Dent Hyg* 1990;64(3):132-8.

6. Shugars DA Miller D, Williams D, Fishburne C, Strickland D. Musculoskeletal pain among general dentists. *Gen Dent* 1987;35:272-6.

7. Kumar C. *Biomechanics in Ergonomics*. Philadelphia: Taylor & Francis 1999:32,233.

8. Chaffin D, Andersson G, Martin B. *Occupational Biomechanics. 3rd ed*. New York: John Wiley & Sons Inc 1999:365-82.

9. Harrison DD, Harrison SO, Croft AC. et al. Sitting Biomechanics Part 1: Review of the Literature. *J Manipulative Physiol Ther* 1999;22:9:594-609.

10. Snijders DJ, Hermans PF, Nieseing R, Spoor CW, Stoeckart R. The influence of slouching and lumbar support on iliolumbar ligaments, intervertebral discs and sacroiliac joints. *Clin Biomech* 2004;19(4):323-9.

11. Calliet R. *Low back pain syndrome. 5th ed*. Philadelphia: F.A. Davis 1995:10,94-143,279.

12. Bogduk N. *Clinical anatomy of the lumbar spine and sacrum. 3rd ed*. Sydney: Churchill Livingstone 1999;101-125, 139.

13. Kroemer K, Grandjean E. *Fitting the task to the human, 5$^{th}$ ed*. Philadelphia: Taylor & Francis 1997:75.

14. Neumann DA. *Kinesiology of the musculoskeletal system. Foundations for physical rehabilitation*. St. Louis: Mosby 2002.

15. Ortengren R, Andersson GB, Nachemson AL. Studies of relationships between lumbar disc pressure, myoelectric back muscle activity, and intra-abdominal (intragastric) pressure. *Spine* 1981;6(1):98-103.

16. Nachemson A. Disc Pressure Measurements. *Spine* 1981;6:93-97.

17. Marklin RW, Cherney K. Working postures of dentists and dental hygienists. *J Calif Dent Assoc* 2005;33(2):133-6.

18. McGill SM. *Low Back Disorders—Evidence-Based Prevention and Rehabilitation*. Champaign, Ill: Human Kinetics 2002:40,51,53-55,116,175, 210-13.

19. Hodges P, Richardson C. Inefficient muscular stabilization of the lumbar spine associated with low back pain: a motor control evaluation of tranverses abdominis. *Spine* 1996;21:2640-50.

20. Hides J, Richardson C. Multifidus muscle recovery is not automatic after resolution of acute, first-episode low back pain. *Spine* 1996;21:2763-9.

21. Richardson C, Jull G, Hodges P, Hides J. *Therapeutic Exercise for Spinal Segmental Stabilization in Low Back Pain.* London, England: J Churchill Livingstone 1999:4-5.

22. Kihara T. Dental care works and work-related complaints of dentists. *Kurume Medical Journal* 1995;42:251-257.

23. Saunders H, Saunders R. *Evaluations, Treatment and Prevention of Musculoskeletal Disorders,* Vol 1. Minnesota: Educational Opportunities, A Saunders Group Company 1995:106.

24. Mandal AC. *The Seated Man: Homo Sedens*. Denmark: Dafnia Publications 1985:28-29.

25. Hokwerda O, Wouters JA, Ruijter RA, Zijlstra-Shaw S. Ergonomic requirements for dental equipment. Guidelines and recommendations for designing, constructing and selecting dental equipment. May 2006. Available at *www.optergo.com/images/Ergonomic_req_april2007.pdf*

26. Bendix T. Adjustment of the seated workplace—with special reference to heights and inclinations of seat and table. *Dan Med Bull* 1987;23(3):125-39.

27. Hedman T, Fernie G. Mechanical response of the lumbar spine to seated postural loads. *Spine* 1997;22:734-743.

28. Williams MM, Hawley JA, McKenzie RA, van Wijmen PM. A comparison of the effects of two sitting postures on back and referred pain. *Spine* 1991; 16(10):1185-91.

29. McGill S, Hughson R, Parks K. Lumbar erector spinae oxygenation during prolonged contractions: implications for prolonged work. *Ergonomics* 2000;43(4):486-93.

30. Lord MJ, Small JM, Dinsay JM, Watkins RG. Lumbar lordosis. Effects of sitting and standing. *Spine* 1997;22(21):2571-4.

31. Callaghan J, McGill S. Low back joint loading and kinematics during standing and unsupported sitting. *Ergonomics* 2001;44(3):280-294.

32. Ratzon N, Yaros M, Kanner T. Musculoskeletal symptoms among dentists in relation to work posture. *Work* 2000; 15:153-158.

33. Toren A. Muscle activity and range of motion during active trunk rotation in a sitting posture. *Applied Ergonomics* 2001;32(6):583-91.

34. Van Dieen J. Asymmetry of erector spinae muscle activity in twisted postures and consistency of muscle activation patterns across subjects. *Spine* 1996;21(22):2651-61.

35. Rundcrantz B, Johnsson B, Moritz U. Occupational cervico-brachial disorders among dentists: Analysis of ergonomics and locomotor functions. *Swed Dent J* 1991;15:105-15.

36. Cailliet R. *Soft Tissue Pain and Disability. 3rd ed*. Philadelphia: F.A. Davis Company 1996:232.

37. Travell JG, Simons DG, Simons LS. Myofascial Pain and Dysfunction: *The Trigger Point Manual, Vol. 1*. Baltimore, Maryland: Lippincott Williams & Wilkins 1999:913-939,613-622;504-537.

38. Hardage JL, Gildersleeve, Rugh JD. Clinical work posture for the dentist: an electromyographic study. *JADA* 1983;107:937-939.

# Chapter Four

1. Lehto TU, Helenius HY, Alaranta HT. Musculoskeletal symptoms of dentists assessed by a multidisciplinary approach. *Community Dent Oral Epidemiol* 1991;19:38-44.

2. Rundcrantz B, Johnsson B, Moritz U. Cervical pain and discomfort among dentists. Epidemiological, clinical and therapeutic aspects. *Swed Dent J* 1990;14:71-80.

3. Murphy D. *Ergonomics and the Dental Care Worker*. Washington, DC: American Public Health Association 1998:381-2.

4. Ariens G, Bongers P, Douwes M, et al. Are neck flexion, neck rotation, and sitting at work risk factors for neck pain? Results of a prospective cohort study. *Occup Environ Med* 2001;58:200-207.

5. Marklin RW, Cherney K. Working Postures of dentists and dental hygienists. *CDA J* 2005;33(2):133-6.

6. Valachi B. Managing Muscles; Neck and shoulder pain among dental hygienists. *Contemp Oral Hyg* 2004;12:12-17.

7. Novak CB, Mackinnon SE. Repetitive Use and Static Postures: a source of nerve compression and pain. *J Hand Ther* 1997;10(2):151-9.

8. Hertling D, Kessler R. *Management of Common Musculoskeletal Disorders. 4th ed*. Philadelphia: Lippincott Williams & Wilkins 2006:741-742.

9. Katevuo K, Aitasalo K, Lehtinen R, Pietila J. Skeletal changes in dentists in Finland. *Dent Oral Epidemiol* 1985;13:23-5.

10. Saunders H, Saunders R. *Evaluations, Treatment and Prevention of Musculoskeletal Disorders,* Vol 1. Minnesota: Educational Opportunities, A Saunders Group Company 1995:6,105.

11. Karwowski W, Marras W. *The Occupational Ergonomics Handbook*. Florida: CRC Press LLC 1999:835.

12. Travell JG, Simons DG, Simons LS. *Myofascial Pain and Dysfunction: The Trigger Point Manual, Vol. 1*. Baltimore, Maryland: Lippincott Williams & Wilkins 1999:278-307,472-83,491-503.

13. Milerad E, Ericson MO, Nisell R, Kilbom A. An electromyographic study of dental work. *Ergonomics* 1991:34(7):953-62.

14. Westgaard R. Effects of physical and mental stressors on muscle pain. *Scand J Work Environ Health* 1999;25(4):19-24.

15. Finsen L, Christensen H, Bakke M. Musculoskeletal disorders among dentists and variation in dental work. *Appl Ergons* 1997;29(2):119-125.

16. Cailliet R. *Neck and Arm Pain. 3rd ed.* Philadelphia: F.A. Davis 1991:59-80.

17. Szeto GP, Straker LM, O'Sullivan PB. A comparison of symptomatic and asymptomatic office workers performing monotonous keyboard work-2: neck and shoulder kinematics. *Man Ther* 2005;10(4):281-91.

18. Branson B, Bray K, Gadbury-Amyot C, et al. Effect of magnification lenses on student operator posture. *J Dent Educ* 2004;68(3):384-89.

19. Falla D, Jull G, Russell T, Vicenzino B, Hodges P. Effect of neck exercise on sitting posture in patients with chronic neck pain. *Phys Ther* 2007; 87(4):408-417.

20. Rundcrantz B, Johnsson B, Moritz U. Occupational cervico-brachial disorders among dentists: Analysis of ergonomics and locomotor functions. *Swed Dent J* 1991;15:105-15.

21. Chaffin D, Andersson G, Martin B. *Occupational Biomechanics. 3rd ed.* New York: John Wiley & Sons Inc 1999;375-85,411.

22. Harris KD, Heer DM, Roy TC, Santos DM, Whitman JM, Wainner RS. Reliability of a measurement of neck flexor muscle endurance. *Phys The* 2005; 85(12):1349-55.

23. Helewa A, Goldsmith CH, Smythe HA, Lee P, Obright K, Stitt LJ. Effect of therapeutic exercise and sleeping neck support on patients with chronic neck pain; a randomized clinical trial. *J Rheumatol* 2007;34(1):151-8.

24. Ferguson LW, Gerwin R. *Clinical Mastery in the Treatment of Myofascial Pain*. Baltimore: Lippincott Williams & Wilkins 2005:2-29.

25. Fernandez-de-las-Penas C, Alonso-Blanco C, Cuadrado ML, Gerwin RD, Pareja JA. Trigger points in the suboccipital muscles and forward head posture in tension-type headache. *Headache* 2006 46(3):454-60.

26. Giuffre K, DiGeronimo TF. *The care and feeding of your brain*. Franklin Lakes: Career Press 1999;160-61.

27. Rains JC, Poceta JS. Headache and sleep disorders: review and clinical implications for headache management. *Headache* 2006;46(9):1344-63.

28. Akesson I, Johnsson B, Rylander L, Moritz U, Skerfving S. Musculoskeletal disorders among female dental personnel – clinical examination and a 5-year follow-up study of symptoms. *Int Arch Occup Environ Health* 1999;72:395-403.

29. Akesson I, Schutz A, Horstmann V, Skerfving S, Moritz U. Musculoskeletal symptoms among dental personnel; – lack of association with mercury and selenium status, overweight and smoking. *Swed Dental J* 2000;24:23-28.
30. Kroemer KHE, Grandjean E. *Fitting The Task To The Human: A Textbook of Occupational Ergonomics. 5th ed.* Philadelphia, Pa: Taylor and Francis; 1997:2,35-45.
31. Valachi B. Balancing your musculoskeletal health. *Woman Dentist Journal* 2004; Nov/Dec:72-76.
32. Sahrmann S. *Diagnosis and Treatment of Movement Impairment Syndromes.* St. Louis: Mosby 2002:21-24.
33. Schuldt K. On neck muscle activity and load reduction in sitting postures. An electromyographic and biomechanical study with applications in ergonomics and rehabilitation. *Scand J Rehab Med Suppl* 1998;19:1-49.
34. Parsell DE, Weber MD, Anderson BC, Cobb GW. Evaluation of Ergonomic dental stools through clinical simulation. *General Dentistry* July/August 2000. 440-444.

# Chapter Five

1. Hamann C, Werner R, Franzblau A, et al. Prevalence of carpal tunnel syndrome and median mononeuropathy among dentists. *J Am Dent Assoc* 2001;132:163-70.
2. Alexopoulos EC, Stathi I, Charizani F. Prevalence of musculoskeletal disorders in dentists. *BMC Musculoskelet Disord* 2004;5:16.
3. Finsen L, Christensen H, Bakke M. Musculoskeletal disorders among dentists and variation in dental work. *Applied Ergonomics* 1997;29(2):119-125.
4. Marshall ED, Duncombe LM, Robinson RQ, Kilbreath, SL. Musculoskeletal symptoms in New South Wales dentists. *Aust Dent J* 1997;42(4):240-6.
5. Rucker LM, Sunell S. Ergonomic Risk Factors Associated with Clinical Dentistry. *CDA J* 2002;30(2):139-48.
6. Lalumandier J, McPhee S. Prevalence and risk factors of hand problems and carpal tunnel syndrome among dental hygienists. *J Dent Hyg* 2001;75:130-133.
7. Akesson I, Johnsson B, Rylander L, Moritz U, Skerfving S. Musculoskeletal disorders among female dental personnel – clinical examination and a 5-year follow-up study of symptoms. *Int Arch Occup Environ Health* 1999;72:395-403.
8. Akesson I, Schutz A, Horstmann V, Skerfving S, Moritz U. Musculoskeletal symptoms among dental personnel; – lack of association with mercury and selenium status, overweight and smoking *Swed Dental J* 2000;24:23-28.
9. Werner R, Hamann C, FranzblauA, Rodgers P. Prevalance of Carpal Tunnel Syndrome and Upper Extremity Tendinitis Among Dental Hygienists. *J Dent Hyg* 2002;76:126-32.
10. Anto C, Aradhya P. Clinical diagnosis of peripheral nerve compression in the upper extremity. *Orthop Clin North Am* 1996;27:227-36.

11. Phalen G. The carpal-tunnel syndrome: seventeen year's experience in diagnosis and treatment of six hundred fifty-four hands. *J Bone Joint Surg Am* 1966;48:221-8.

12. Mackin EJ, Callahan AD, Osterman AL, Skirven TM, Schneider LH. *Rehabilitation of the hand and upper extremity, 4th ed.* St. Louis: Mosby 2002:644-667.

13. Karwowski W, Marras WS. *The Occupational Ergonomics Handbook.* Boca Raton, Florida: CRC Press 1999:775-777,821-825,1643-44.

14. Rice VJ, Nindel B, Pentikis JS. Dental Workers, Musculoskeletal Cumulative Trauma, and Carpal Tunnel Syndrome: Who is at Risk? A Pilot Study. *Int J Occup Saf Ergon* 1996;2(3):218-233.

15. Cailliet R. *Neck and Arm Pain. 3rd ed.* Philadelphia: F.A. Davis 1991; 195-197,212,215-218.

16. Whyte-Ferguson L, Gerwin R. *Clinical mastery in the treatment of myofascial pain.* Philadelphia: Lippincott Williams & Wilkins 2005;145-166.

17. Chin DH, Jones NF. Repetitive Motion Hand Disorders. *CDA J* 2002; 30(2):149-160.

18. Ericson, WB. Median Nerve Entrapment in the Forearm: Diagnosis and Treatment, Poster Presentation, American Society for Surgery of the Hand, 59th Annual Meeting, N.Y.C., 2004.

19. Feldman, RG, Goldman R, and Keyserling, WM. Peripheral nerve entrapment syndromes and ergonomic factors. *Am J Ind Med* 1983;4(5):661-81.

20. Occupational disease surveillance: carpal tunnel syndrome. *MMWR (Morbidity and Mortality Weekly Report)* 1989;18:36-44.

21. Dong H, Barr A, Loomer P, Rempel D. The effects of finger rest positions on hand muscle load and pinch force in simulated dental hygiene work. *J Dent Educ* 2005;69(4):453-60.

22. Pattison AM, Matsuda S, Pattison GL. Extraoral fulcrums; the essentials of using extraoral fulcrums for periodontal instrumentation. *Dimensions of dental hygiene* 2004;2(10):20, 21-23.

23. Matsuda S. Technique – Proper Grasp. *Dimensions of dental hygiene* 2005; 3(9):26,28.

23. Matsuda S. Troubleshooting technique – sharpening. *Dimensions of dental hygiene* 2005;3(6):32,34.

24. Matsuda S. Instrumentation of Biofilm. *Dimensions of dental hygiene.* 2003;1(1):26-28, 30.

25. Morse TF, Michalak-Turcotte C, Atwood-Sanders M, Warren N, Paterson DR, Bruneau H, Cherniack M. A pilot study of hand and arm musculoskeletal disorders in dental hygiene students. *J Dent Hyg* 2003;77(30):173-9.

26. Dong H, Barr A, Loomer P, LaRoche C, Young E, Rempel D. The effects of periodontal instrument handle design on hand muscle load and pinch force, *J Am Dent Assoc* 2006;137(8):1123-30.

27. Simmer-Beck M, Bray KK, Branson B, Glaros A, Weeks J. Comparision of muscle activity associated with structural differences in dental hygiene mirrors. *J Dent Hyg* 2006;80(1):8.

28. Glasscoe D. The better way to sharpen dental instruments – CD. *Professional Dental Management Inc.* 2006.

29. Kumar C. *Biomechanics in Ergonomics*. Philadelphia: Taylor & Francis 1999:165-175.

30. Stockstill JW, Harn SD, Stickland D, Hruska R. Prevalence of upper extremity neuropathy in a clinical dentist population. *J Am Dent Assoc* 1993;124:67-72.

31. Weiss S, Falkenstein N. *Hand rehabilitation; a quick reference guide and review, 2nd ed.* St. Louis: Elsevier Mosby 2005;346.

32. Travell JG, Simons DG, Simons LS. *Myofascial Pain and Dysfunction: The Trigger Point Manual, Vol. 1.* Baltimore, Maryland: Lippincott Williams & Wilkins 1999.

33. Novak CB, Mackinnon SE. Repetitive Use and Static Postures: a source of nerve compression and pain. *J Hand Ther* 1997;10(2):151-9.

34. Adelman S, Eisner K. Arm pain in a dentist: pronator syndrome. *J Am Dent Assoc* 1982;105:61-62.

35. Valachi B, Valachi K. Mechanisms contributing to musculoskeletal disorders in dentistry. *J Am Dent Assoc* 2003;134:1344-50.

36. Ritter A, Sensat M, Harn, S. Thoracic Outlet Syndrome: A review of the literature. *J Dent Hyg* 1999;73:205-7.

37. Powell BJ, Winkley GP, Brown JO, Etersque S. Evaluating the fit of ambidextrous and fitted gloves: Implications for hand discomfort. *J Am Dent Assoc* 1994;125:1235-42.

38. Christensen G. Operating gloves: The good and the bad. *J Am Dent Assoc* 2001;132:1455-57.

39. Hwang M, Kang YK, Shin jY, Kim DH: Referred pain pattern of the abductor pollicis longus muscle. *Am J Phy Med Rehabil* 2005;84:593-597.

40. Milerad E, Ericson MO, Nisell R, Kilbom A. An Electromyographic study of Dental work. *Ergonomics* 1991:34:953-962.

# Chapter Six

1. Rising DW, Bennett BC, Hursh K, Plesh O. Reports of body pain in a dental student population. *JADA* 2005;136:81-86.

2. Morse T, Bruneau H, Michalak-Turcotte C, Sanders M, Warren N, Dussetschleger J, Diva U, Croteau M, Cherniack M. Musculoskeletal disorders of the neck and shoulder in dental hygienists and dental hygiene students. *J Dent Hyg* 2007;81(1):10.

3. White S. Ergonomics: How does dentistry fit you? *Woman Dentist Journal* Jan 2003.

4.  Harrison DD, Harrison SO, Croft AC. et al. Sitting Biomechanics Part 1: Review of the Literature. *J Manipulative Physiol Ther* 1999;22:9:594-609.

5.  Karwowski W, Marras W. *The Occupational Ergonomics Handbook.* Florida: CRC Press LLC 1999:1765-66,185,219.

6.  Snijders DJ, Hermans PF, Nieseing R, Spoor CW, Stoeckart R. The influence of slouching and lumbar support on iliolumbar ligaments, intervertebral discs and sacroiliac joints. *Clin Biomech* 2004;19(4):323-9.

7.  Kumar C. *Biomechanics in Ergonomics.* Philadelphia: Taylor & Francis 1999:32,233.

8.  McGill SM. *Low Back Disorders—Evidence-Based Prevention and Rehabilitation.* Champaign, Ill: Human Kinetics 2002;175-7.

9.  Valachi B, Valachi K. Operator Seating: The tall and short of it. *Dent Today* 2005;1:108-110.

10. Chaffin D, Andersson G, Martin B. *Occupational Biomechanics. 3rd ed.* New York: John Wiley & Sons Inc 1999;113,365-82.

11. Williams MM, Hawley JA, McKenzie RA, van Wijmen PM. A comparison of the effects of two sitting postures on back and referred pain. *Spine* 1991; 16(10):1185-91.

12. Parsell DE, Weber MD, Anderson BC, Cobb GW. Evaluation of Ergonomic dental stools through clinical simulation. *Gent Dent* 2000;48(4):440-4.

13. Schuldt K, Ekholm J, Harms-Ringdahl K, Nemeth G, Arborelius UP. Effects of arm support of suspension on neck and shoulder muscle activity during sedentary work. *Scand J Rehabil Med* 1987;19(2):77-84.

14. Schuldt K. On neck muscle activity and load reduction in sitting postures. An electromyographic and biomechanical study with applications in ergonomics and rehabilitation. *Scand J Rehab Med Suppl* 1998;19:1-49.

15. Ahearn D. The 8 Keys to selecting great seating for long-term health. *Dent Today* 2005;24(9):128,130-1.

16. Hokwerda O, Wouters JA, Ruijter RA, Zijlstra-Shaw S. Ergonomic requirements for dental equipment. Guidelines and recommendations for designing, constructing and selecting dental equipment. May 2006. Available at: *www.optergo.com/images/Ergonomic_req_april2007.pdf*

17. Spear F. One clinician's journey through the use of magnification in dentistry. *Advanced Esthetics and Interdisciplinary Dentistry* 2006;2(4):30-33.

18. Cuomo GM. Posture-Directed vs. Image-Directed Dentistry: Ergonomic and Economic Advantages Through Dental Microscope Use. *Sidekick: Equipment Technology & News For You and Your Dental Practice.* 2006; Summer:42-46.

19. Nase JB. Clinical operating microscopes: They're not just for endodontists anymore. *Pa Dent J* 2005;72(5):30-3.

20. Nase JB. The clinical operating microscope advantage in fixed prosthodontics. *Gen Dent* 2003;51(5):417-22.

21. Branson B, Bray K, Gadbury-Amyot C, et al. Effect of magnification lenses on student operator posture. *J Dent Educ* 2004;68(3):384-9.

22. Chang BJ. Ergonomic Benefits of Surgical Telescope Systems: Selection Guidelines. *CDA J* 2002;30(2)161-9.

23. Cailliet R. *Neck and Arm Pain. 3rd ed.* Philadelphia: F.A. Davis 1991;74-75.

24. Rucker L, Beattie C, McGregor C, Sunell S, Ito Y. Declination angle and its role in selecting surgical telescopes. *J Am Dent Assoc* 1999;130:1096-100.

25. Valachi B. Vision Quest: Finding your best working distance when using loupes. *Dental Practice Report* 2006;4:49-50.

26. Kroemer K, Grandjean E. *Fitting the task to the human, 5th ed.* Philadelphia:Taylor & Francis 1997;295-317.

27. Matsuda S. Troubleshooting technique – sharpening. *Dimensions of dental hygiene* 2005;3(6):32,34.

28. Glasscoe D. The better way to sharpen dental instruments – CD. Professional Dental Management Inc. 2006.

29. Powell BJ, Winkley GP, Brown JO, Etersque S. Evaluating the fit of ambidextrous and fitted gloves: Implications for hand discomfort. *J Am Dent Assoc* 1994;125:1235-1242.

# Chapter Seven

1. An Introduction to Ergonomics: Risk Factors, MSDs, Approaches and Interventions. A report of the Ergonomics and Disability Support Advisory Committee (EDSAC) to Council on Dental Practice: American Dental Association 2004:18. Available at: *www.ada.org/prof/prac/wellness/ergonomics_paper.pdf* Accessed September 15, 2007.

2. O'Brien D. Phone interview with equipment specialist for Burkhart Dental Supply on January 30, 2007.

3. Toren A. Muscle activity and range of motion during active trunk rotation in a sitting posture. *Applied Ergonomics* 2001;32(6):583-91.

4. Van Dieen J. Asymmetry of erector spinae muscle activity in twisted postures and consistency of muscle activation patterns across subjects. *Spine* 1996;21(22):2651-61.

5. Valachi B. Can delivery systems deliver pain? *Dental Practice Report* 2006; 6:60-62.

6. Ahearn, David. Ten essential elements of a productive treatment room – Part 1. *Dent Econ* 2002; June.

7. Kroemer K, Grandjean E. *Fitting the task to the human, 5th ed.* Philadelphia, PA: Taylor & Francis 1997;55-56,66-68.

8. Ahearn D. One dozen essential elements of a great office design – Part 2. *Dent Econ* 2002; May.

9. Lavine L. Technology in the Dental Office: Ergonomic Considerations. *www.thedigitaldentist.com/index/use_lang/EN/page/152/cnt_id/91.html* Accessed on 05/01/07.

10. Fetzer M. Interview with President of Dental Systems Integrators Inc. on September 9, 2007.

11. Ahearn, David. The Ergonomic Conundrum for Technology Integration. *Alpha Omegan* 2006; December:110-112.

# Chapter Eight

1. Calliet R. *Low back pain syndrome. 5th ed.* Philadelphia: F.A. Davis; 1995:179.

2. Shugars DA, Miller D, Williams D, Fishburne C, Strickland D. Musculoskeletal pain among general dentists. *Gen Dent* 1987;35:272-6.

3. Osborn JB, Newell KJ, Rudney JD, Stoltenberg JL. Musculoskeletal pain among Minnesota dental hygienists. *J Dent Hyg* 1990;64(3):132-8.

4. Lehto TU, Helenius HY, Alaranta HT. Musculoskeletal symptoms of dentists assessed by a multidisciplinary approach. *Community Dent Oral Epidemiol* 1991;19:38-44.

5. Rundcrantz B, Johnsson B, Moritz U. Occupational cervico-brachial disorders among dentists: Analysis of ergonomics and locomotor functions. *Swed Dent J* 1991;15:105-15.

6. Travell JG, Simons DG, Simons LS. *Myofascial Pain and Dysfunction: The Trigger Point Manual, Vol. 1.* Baltimore, Maryland: Lippincott Williams & Wilkins 1999;111,179-87.

7. Fernandez-de-las-Penas C, Alonso-Blanco C, Cuadrado ML, Gerwin RD, Pareja JA. Trigger points in the suboccipital muscles and forward head posture in tension-type headache. *Headache* 2006 Mar;46(3):454-60.

8. Gerwin RD. Classification, epidemiology, and natural history of myofascial pain syndrome. *Curr Pain Headache Rep* 2001;5(5):412-20.

9. Hanten W, Olson S, Butts N, Nowicki A. Effectiveness of a Home Program of Ischemic Pressure Followed by Sustained Stretch for Treatment of Myofascial Trigger Points. *Physical Therapy* 2000;80,997-1003.

10. Cherkin DC, Sherman KJ, Deyo RA, Shekelle PG. A review of the evidence of the effectiveness, safety, and cost of acupuncture, massage therapy, and spinal manipulation for back pain. *Ann Intern Med* 2003;138(11):898-906.

# Chapter Nine

1. Miranda H, Viikari-Juntura E, Martikainen R, Takala EP, Riihimaki H. A prospective study of work related factors and physical exercise as predictors of shoulder pain. *Occup Environ Med* 2001;58(8):528-34.

2. Linton SJ, van Tulder MW. Preventive interventions for back and neck pain problems: what is the evidence? *Spine* 2001;26(7):778-87.

3. Kay TM, Gross A, Goldsmith C, Santaguida PL, et al. Exercises for mechanical neck disorders. *Cochrane Database Syst Rev* 2005;(3):CD004250.

4. Vasseljen O Jr, Johansen BM, Westgaard RH. The effect of pain reduction on perceived tension and EMG-recorded trapezius muscle activity in workers with shoulder and neck pain. *Scand J Rehab Med* 1995;27(4):243-52.

5. Lehto TU, Helenius HY, Alaranta HT. Musculoskeletal symptoms of dentists assessed by a multidisciplinary approach. *Community Dent Oral Epidemiol* 1991;19:38-44.

6. Bassett S. Back problems among dentists. *J Can Dent Assoc* 1983; 49(4):251-6.

7. Shugars DA Miller D, Williams D, Fishburne C, Strickland D. Musculoskeletal pain among general dentists. *Gen Dent* 1987;35:272-6.

8. Osborn JB, Newell KJ, Rudney JD, Stoltenberg JL. Musculoskeletal pain among Minnesota dental hygienists. *J Dent Hyg* 1990;64(3):132-8.

9. Lehto TU, Helenius HY, Alaranta HT. Musculoskeletal symptoms of dentists assessed by a multidisciplinary approach. *Community Dent Oral Epidemiol* 1991;19:38-44.

10. Rundcrantz B, Johnsson B, Moritz U. Occupational cervico-brachial disorders among dentists: Analysis of ergonomics and locomotor functions. *Swed Dent J* 1991;15:105-15.

11. Valachi B, Valachi K. Mechanisms contributing to musculoskeletal disorders in dentistry. *J Am Dent Assoc* 2003;134(10):1344-50.

12. Valachi B. Compromising positions. Exercises that can improve or worsen dentist's musculoskeletal health. *Dental Practice Report* 2005; 5:8-12.

13. Thacker SB, Gilchrist J, Stroup DF, Kimsey CD. The impact of stretching on sports injury risk: a systematic review of the literature. *Med Sci Sports Exerc* 2004:36(3):371-8.

14. Bauman AE. Updating the evidence that physical activity is good for health: an epidemiological review 2000-2003. *J Sci Med Sport* 2004;7(1 Suppl): 6-19.

15. Blair SN, Kohl HW 3rd, Paffenbarger RS Jr, Clark DG, Cooper KH, Gibbons LW. Physical fitness and all-cause mortality. A prospective study of healthy men and women. *J Am Dent Assoc* 1989;262(17):2395-401.

16. Villenueve PJ, Morrison HI, Craig CL, Schaubel DE. Physical activity, physical fitness, and risk of dying. *Epidemiology* 1998; 9(6):626-31.

17. McGill S. *Low Back Disorders: Evidence-Based Prevention and Rehabilitation*. Champaign, Ill: Human Kinetics 2002;100-1,177,253.

18. Baechle T, Earle R. *Essentials of Strength Training and Conditioning. 2nd Ed*. Champaign, Ill: Human Kinetics 2000;64-66.

19. Magnusson SP. Passive properties of human skeletal muscle during stretch maneuvers. A review. *Scand J Med Sci Sports* 1998;8(2):65-77.

20. O'Sullivan PB, Mitchell T, Bulich P, Holte J. The relationship between posture and back muscle endurance in industrial workers with flexion-related low back pain. *Manual Therapy* 2006;11(4):264-71.

21. McArdle W, Katch F, Katch V. *Exercise Physiology:Energy, Nutrition and Human Performance 5th ed.* Philadelphia: Lippincott Williams and Wilkins 2001.
22. Norkin CC, Levangie PK. *Joint structure and function. A comprehensive analysis, 4th ed.* Philadelphia: F.A. Davis Company 2005.
23. Jones AC, Forsythe S. Functional training for dentistry: An exercise prescription for dental healthcare personnel. *CDA J* 2005;33(2):137-45.
24. Souza G, Baker L, Powers C. Electromyographic activity of selected trunk muscles during dynamic spine stabilization exercises. *Arch Phys Med Rehab* 2001;82(11):1551-7.
25. Shamus E, Shamus J. *Sports Injury Prevention & Rehabilitation.* New York: Mcgraw Hill 2001;185-239.
26. Valachi B. Par for the course. Dentists, golf and low back pain. *Dental Practice Report* 2007;3:11-14.
27. Lindsay D, Horton J. Comparison of spine motion in elite golfers with and without low back pain. *J Sports Sci* 2002;20(8):599-605.
28. Evans C, Oldreive W. A study to investigate whether golfers with a history of low back pain show a reduced endurance of the transversus abdominus. *The Journal of Manual and Manipulative Therapy* 2000;8(4):162-74.
29. Grimshaw P, Giles A, Tong R, Grimmer K. Lower back and elbow injuries in golf. *Sports Med* 2002;32(10):655-66.
30. Kihara T. Dental care works and work-related complaints of dentists. *Kurume Medical Journal.* 1995;42:251-257.
31. Van Dieen J. Asymmetry of erector spinae muscle activity in twisted postures and consistency of muscle activation patterns across subjects. *Spine* 1996;21(22):2651-61.
32. Egler T. Pilates Precautions. *Physical Therapy Products* 2006; June:20-22.

# Chapter Ten

1. Martin P. *The Healing Mind.* New York: St. Martin's Griffin 1999;174,176, 197,212,247-8.
2. Westgaard R. Effects of physical and mental stressors on muscle pain. *Scand J Work and Environ Health* 1999;25(4):19-24.
3. Holte KA, Westgaard RH. Daytime trapezius muscle activity and shoulder-neck pain of service workers with work stress and low biomechanical exposure. *Am J Ind Med* 2002;41(5):393-405.
4. Hertling D, Kessler R. *Management of Common Musculoskeletal Disorders. 4th ed.* Philadelphia: Lippincott Williams & Wilkins 2006;140-60.
5. Freeman R, Main JR, Burke FJ. Occupational stress and dentistry: theory and practice. Part II. Assessment and control. *Br Dent J* 1995;178(6):218-22.
6. Rada RE, Johnson-Leong C. Stress, burnout, anxiety and depression among dentists. J Am Dent Assoc 2004;135(6):788-94.

7. Gorter RC, Albrecht G, Hoogstraten J, Eijkman MA. Measuring work stress among Dutch dentists. *Int Dent J* 1999;49(3):144-52.

8. O'Shea RM, Corah NL, Ayer WA. Sources of dentists' stress. *J Am Dent Assoc* 1984;109(1):48-51.

9. Lehto TU, Helenius HY, Alaranta HT. Musculoskeletal symptoms of dentists assessed by a multidisciplinary approach. *Community Dent Oral Epidemiol* 1991;19:38-44.

10. Newton JT, Allen CD, Coates J, Turner A, Prior J. How to reduce the stress of general dental practice: the need for research into the effectiveness of multifaceted interventions. *Br Dent J* 2006;200(8):437-40.

11. Moore R, Brodsgaard I. Dentists' perceived stress and its relation to perceptions about anxious patients. *Community Dent Oral Epidemiol* 2001;29(1):73-80.

12. Pohlmann K, Jonas I, Ruf S, Harzer W. Stress, burnout and health in the clinical period of dental education. *Eur J Dent Educ* 2005;9(2):78-84.

13. Alaujan AH, Alzahem AM. Stress among dentists. *Gen Dent* 2004; 52(5): 428-32.

14. Burke FJ, Main JR, Freeman R. The practice of dentistry: an assessment of reasons for premature retirement. *Br Dent J* 1997;182(7):250-4.

15. Rundcrantz B, Johnsson B, Moritz U, Roxendal G. Occupational cervico-brachial disorders among dentists. Psychosocial work environment, personal harmony and life-satisfaction. *Scand J Soc Med* 1991;19(3):174-80.

16. Gorter RC. Work stress and burnout among dental hygienists. *Int J Dent Hyg* 2005;3(2):88-92.

17. Ylipaa V, Arnetz BB, Preber H. Factors that affect health and well-being in dental hygienists; a comparison of Swedish dental practices. *J Dent Hyg* 1999;73(4):191-9.

18. Wilson RF, Coward PY, Capewell J, Laidler TL, Rigby AC, Shaw TJ. Perceived sources of occupational stress in general dental practitioners. *Br Dent J* 1998;23;184(10):499-502.

19. Miles L. *Dynamic Dentistry: Practice management tools and strategy for breakthrough success.* Virginia Beach: Link Publishing 2003;89-109.

20. Dower JS Jr, Simon JF, Peltier B, Chambers D. Patients who make a dentist most anxious about giving injections. *J Calif Dent Assoc* 1995;23(9):35-40.

21. Ylipaa V, Arnetz BB, Benko, SS, Ryden H. Physical and psychosocial work environments among Swedish dental hygienists: risk indicators for musculoskeletal complaints. *Swed Dent J* 1997;21(3)111-20.

22. Ylipaa V, Arnetz BB, Preber H, Benko SS. Determinants of work satisfaction among Swedish dental hygienists. *Scand J Caring Sci* 1996;10(4):247-53.

23. Rutter H, Herzberg J, Paice E. Stress in doctors and dentists who teach. *Med Educ* 2002;36(6):543-9.

24. Davis M, Eshelman E, Mckay M. *The Relaxation & Stress Reduction Workbook, 5th ed.* Oakland, Calif.: New Harbinger Publications 2000.

25. Sklar D. Stressed out? Relax and Read On. *Doctor of Dentistry* 2004;4:15-17.

26. Bost N, Wallis M. The effectiveness of a 15 minute weekly massage in reducing physical and psychological stress in nurses. *Aust J Adv Nurs* 2006; 23(4):28-33.

27. Long L, Huntley A, Ernst E. Which complementary and alternative therapies benefit which conditions? A survey of the opinions of 223 professional organizations. *Complement Ther Med* 2001;9(3):178-85.

28. Peterson C et al. Pessimistic explanatory style is a risk factor for physical illness: a thirty-five-year longitudinal study. *J Pers Soc Psychol* 1988;55(1):23-7.

# Chapter Eleven

1. Murphy D. *Ergonomics and the Dental Care Worker.* Washington, D.C.: American Public Health Association 1998;151-153.

2. Lalumandier J, McPhee S, Parrott C, Vendemia M. Musculoskeletal pain: prevalence, prevention, and differences among dental office personnel. *Gen Dent* 2001;49:150-6.

3. Valachi B. *The ergonomics of dental assisting: Preventing and managing work-related pain.* Chicago: American Dental Assistant's Association: Department of Continuing Education 2004.

4. Chaffin D, Andersson G, Martin B. *Occupational Biomechanics.* 3rd ed. New York: John Wiley & Sons Inc. 1999:375-85,411.

5. Van Dieen J. Asymmetry of erector spinae muscle activity in twisted postures and consistency of muscle activation patterns across subjects. *Spine* 1996;21(22):2651-61.

6. Toren A. Muscle activity and range of motion during active trunk rotation in a sitting posture. *Applied Ergonomics* 2001;32(6):583-91.

7. Valachi B. *Fighting Plaque with a Healthy Back.* Lecture presented at: American Dental Assistant Association National Convention. July 15, 2005. Washington, D.C.

8. Callaghan J, McGill S. Low back joint loading and kinematics during standing and unsupported sitting. *Ergonomics* 2001;44(3):280-294.

9. Ratzon NZ, Yaros T, Mizlik A, Kanner T. Musculoskeletal symptoms among dentists in relation to work posture. *Work* 2000;15:153-8.

10. Akesson I, Johnsson B, Rylander L, Moritz U, Skerfving S. Musculoskeletal disorders among female dental personnel – clinical examination and a 5-year follow-up study of symptoms. *Int Arch Occup Environ Health* 1999;72:395-403.

11. Whyte-Ferguson L, Gerwin R. *Clinical mastery in the treatment of myofascial pain.* Philadelphia: Lippincott Williams & Wilkins 2005:145-166.

# Chapter Twelve

1. Valachi B. Front Desk: Pain Prevention. *Dental Practice Report* 2006;5:13-20.

2. IJmker S, Blatter BM, van der beek AJ, van Mechelen W, Bongers PM. Prospective research on musculoskeletal disorders in office workers (PROMO):study protocol. *BMC Musculoskelet Disord* 2006;5(7):55.

3. Damany S, Bellis J. *It's not carpal tunnel syndrome! RSI theory and therapy for computer professionals*. Philadelphia: Simax 2000.

4. Chaffin D, Andersson G, Martin B. *Occupational Biomechanics. 3rd ed.* New York: John Wiley & Sons Inc 1999:365-82.

5. Kroemer K, Grandjean E. *Fitting the task to the human, 5th ed.* Philadelphia: Taylor & Francis;1997:53-100.

6. Karwowski W, Marras W. *The Occupational Ergonomics Handbook*. Florida: CRC Press LLC 1999:1765-66.

7. Working safely with video display terminals. McLean L, Tingley M, Scott R, Richards J. Computer terminal work and the benefit of microbreaks. *Applied Ergonomics* 2001;32:225-237

# Index

## A

anti-inflammatory drugs, 132
armrests
   benefits of, 70
   selection and adjustment, 98-99
assistant delivery systems, 123–124, 189-190
assistant mobile carts, *123*, 190
assistant, dental
   delivery systems, 123-124,189–190
   posture and movement concerns, 182–183, 187–188
   standing, 189
   stool features and adjustment, 183–187
author information, 239

## B

back disorders. *See also* low back pain
   risk factors for, 45-52
   upper back pain, 51
bibliography, 219-238

## C

carpal tunnel
   anatomy, 77–79
   illustration, 77
carpal tunnel pressure
   forceful pinch grip and, 78, 82
   instrument diameter and, 81
carpal tunnel syndrome (CTS)
   defined, 7, 76–77
   diagnosis, 83–85
   pain syndromes that mimic, 85–88
   prevalence of, 75-76
   risk factors for, 78-79
   symptoms, 78-79, 84
   treatment, 83–85

carpal tunnel syndrome (CTS) prevention strategies
   cord management, 83
   grip pressure reduction, 82
   instrument selection, 80–82
   stretching, 43, 83
   switching hands, 82
   temperature, 83
   wrist posture, 79-80
certified neuromuscular therapist, (CNMT), 86, 135
certified hand therapist (CHT), 135
cervical instability, 64–65
cervical radicular pain, 87
chairs
   ergonomic features of 100-101
   orientation, 125
chairside stretches, 39-43
chiropractors, 135
chronic pain, 138–141
clock positions, in relation to patient chair, 35-36, 56-57
computer ergonomics in front office, 196–200
computer technology in operatory, 125–127
cord management, 83
counter and delivery system height, 122–123
cumulative trauma disorders (CTDs), 4
   common types in dentistry, 6–7
   in dental assistants, 182
   financial impact of, 4-6
   in front office, 194
   risk factors leading to, 8–9

## D

de Quervain's syndrome, 76, 88–89
delivery systems, 116–121
dental assistants
   delivery systems, 123-124,189–190

# About the Author

Bethany Valachi is a physical therapist, dental ergonomic consultant and president of *Posturedontics®*, a company that provides research-based dental ergonomic education and evaluates dental products. She is clinical instructor of ergonomics at OHSU School of Dentistry in Portland, Oreg., and has provided expertise on dental ergonomics to faculty and students at numerous dental universities and hygiene schools, including faculty training at New York University College of Dentistry. As a certified ergonomic assessment specialist, she also consults with practicing dental professionals to improve ergonomics, work more comfortably and extend their careers with preventive strategies both in and outside the operatory.

A member of the National Speaker's Association, Bethany lectures internationally at dental study clubs, state associations and national dental meetings. She is widely published in the *Journal of the American Dental Association (JADA), Australian Dental Practice, Contemporary Oral Hygiene* and numerous other peer-reviewed dental journals. Bethany is author of the *ADAA Ergonomic Home Study Course* and has produced chairside stretching and home exercise videos specifically for dental professionals. She lives in Portland, Oregon with her husband, Dr. Keith Valachi, who operates a private dental practice in St. Helens, Oreg.

She was prompted to write this book due to numerous requests from dental professionals in search of the secrets to a pain-free practice. Bethany is now sharing this with you—the comfortable side of dentistry.

# posturedontics®

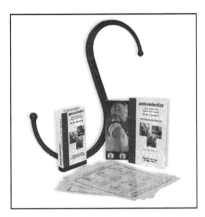
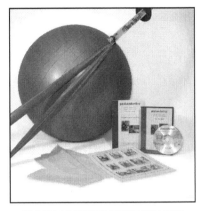

# QUICK ORDER FORM

## FOUR EASY WAYS TO ORDER:

**Fax:** Fax this form to (503) 291-1678
**Online:** www.posturedontics.com
**Phone:** (503) 291-5121
**Mail:** Send this form to Posturedontics,
P.O. Box 25552, Portland, OR 97298

**DENTISTS:**
Earn AGD
PACE credits
with DVD kits!

## PLEASE SEND MORE FREE INFORMATION ON:

❏ Additional Products
❏ In-Office Ergonomic Counseling

❏ Scheduling a Seminar
❏ Upcoming Seminars

❏ Please add me to your
electronic newsletter

Name:_____ Email (required): _____

Address:_____ City: _____
*(Must match billing address of credit card)*

State:_____ ZIP:_____ Height:_____ (required for Exercise Package)

Payment Method:  ❏ MC  ❏ VISA  ❏ Discover  ❏ Check (add $10 for S/H)

Credit Card Number:_____ Exp.: _____

Signature _____

| QUANTITY | ITEM | COST* |
|---|---|---|
| | *Practice Dentistry Pain-Free* Book—B. Valachi | $39.95 |
| VHS _____  DVD _____  *(indicate your height)* | *Smart Moves* Home Exercise *DVD Kit for Dental Professionals includes:*<br>• *On the Ball* Exercise videotape or DVD<br>• Swiss Exercise Ball<br>• 2 plugs and bicycle pump adapter<br>• 2 elastic exercise bands and door anchor<br>• Exercise instruction manual and cue card | $129.95 |
| VHS _____  DVD _____ | *Smart Moves* Chairside Stretching *DVD Kit includes:*<br>• *Chairside Stretching* videotape or DVD<br>• Set of three laminated stretching wall charts<br>• Chairside stretching instruction manual<br>• Backnobber trigger point tool and user guide | $129.95 |
| VHS ___ DVD ___ | **Order BOTH DVD Kits (Save $70.00)** | **$189.95** |

*\* In USD plus shipping. Prices are as of book printing date and subject to change.*

*Office Use Only:*   Date:        Wt:        Ft:        Total:        Auth. #

# posturedontics®

## PAIN AND INJURY PREVENTION
## PRODUCTS FOR DENTAL CARE WORKERS

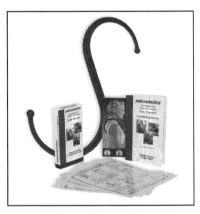

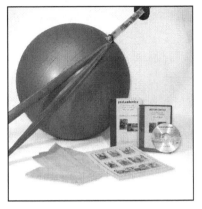

### CHAIRSIDE STRETCHING AND TRIGGER POINT THERAPY KIT
(VHS or DVD)

Prevent or reverse the progression of chronic work-related pain with 19 stretching techniques specifically designed for dentists and hygienists to use during their workday. Plus self-treat painful trigger points. Kit includes:

- 30-minute VHS/DVD
- 3 laminated stretching wall charts
- Backnobber massage tool
- 19 illustrations
- Instruction booklet

The DVD is excellent for team meetings and study clubs.

**$129.95**

### SMART MOVES EXERCISE KIT
(VHS or DVD)

We've fused Pilates, physical therapy and dental ergonomics into a fun, low-impact exercise routine that helps dental professionals prevent or reverse chronic pain syndromes. Using a Swiss exercise ball and Theraband, you'll strengthen and balance key muscle groups and increase your flexibility in problem areas. You will also learn which exercises can worsen dental professionals' health. Kit includes:

- 25-minute exercise VHS/DVD
- Swiss Ball
- Theraband
- Door anchor
- Exercise cue card

**$129.95**

## SAVE $70
### WHEN YOU ORDER BOTH DVD KITS!
## A $260 VALUE FOR $189.95

# QUICK ORDER FORM

## FOUR EASY WAYS TO ORDER:

**Fax:** Fax this form to (503) 291-1678
**Online:** www.posturedontics.com
**Phone:** (503) 291-5121
**Mail:** Send this form to Posturedontics,
P.O. Box 25552, Portland, OR 97298

*DENTISTS: Earn AGD PACE credits with DVD kits!*

## PLEASE SEND MORE FREE INFORMATION ON:

❑ Additional Products
❑ In-Office Ergonomic Counseling
❑ Scheduling a Seminar
❑ Upcoming Seminars
❑ Please add me to your electronic newsletter

Name:_____ Email (required): _____

Address:_____ City: _____
*(Must match billing address of credit card)*

State:_____ ZIP:_____ Height:_____ (required for Exercise Package)

Payment Method: ❑ MC ❑ VISA ❑ Discover ❑ Check (add $10 for S/H)

Credit Card Number:_____ Exp.: _____

Signature _____

| QUANTITY | ITEM | COST* |
|---|---|---|
| | *Practice Dentistry Pain-Free* Book—B. Valachi | $39.95 |
| VHS _____<br><br>DVD _____<br><br>*(indicate your height)* | *Smart Moves* Home Exercise *DVD Kit for Dental Professionals includes:*<br>• *On the Ball* Exercise videotape or DVD<br>• Swiss Exercise Ball<br>• 2 plugs and bicycle pump adapter<br>• 2 elastic exercise bands and door anchor<br>• Exercise instruction manual and cue card | $129.95 |
| VHS _____<br><br>DVD _____ | *Smart Moves* Chairside Stretching *DVD Kit includes:*<br>• *Chairside Stretching* videotape or DVD<br>• Set of three laminated stretching wall charts<br>• Chairside stretching instruction manual<br>• Backnobber trigger point tool and user guide | $129.95 |
| VHS ___ DVD ___ | **Order BOTH DVD Kits (Save $70.00)** | **$189.95** |

*\* In USD plus shipping. Prices are as of book printing date and subject to change.*

*Office Use Only:* Date: Wt: Ft: Total: Auth. #